PLATINUM VIGNETTES™

ULTRA-HIGH-YIELD CLINICAL CASE SCENARIOS FOR USMLE STEP 2

Internal Medicine

ESR
ANA
RF
TSH

PLATINUM VIGNETTES™

ULTRA-HIGH-YIELD CLINICAL CASE SCENARIOS
FOR USMLE STEP 2

Internal Medicine

ADAM BROCHERT, MD
Resident
Department of Radiology
Medical College of Georgia
Memorial Health University Medical Center
Savannah, Georgia

Hanley & Belfus, Inc. / Philadelphia

Publisher: HANLEY & BELFUS, INC.
Medical Publishers
210 South 13th Street
Philadelphia, PA 19107
(215) 546-7293; 800-962-1892
FAX (215) 790-9330
Web site: http://www.hanleyandbelfus.com

Note to the reader: Although the information in this book has been carefully reviewed for correctness of dosage and indications, neither the author nor the publisher can accept any legal responsibility for any errors or omissions that may be made. Neither the publisher nor the author makes any warranty, expressed or implied, with respect to the material contained herein. Before prescribing any drug, the reader must review the manufacturer's current product information (package inserts) for accepted indications, absolute dosage recommendations, and other information pertinent to the safe and effective use of the product described. This is especially important when drugs are given in combination or as an adjunct to other forms of therapy.

PLATINUM VIGNETTES™: INTERNAL MEDICINE ISBN 1-56053-531-8

Library of Congress Control Number: 2002102750

Last digit is the print number: 9 8 7 6 5 4 3 2 1

INTRODUCTION

Case scenarios are a great way to review for the USMLE Step 2 exam. A high percentage of current exam questions center on case studies or patient presentations in an office or emergency department setting. Practicing this format and being familiar with the majority of the classic, "guaranteed-to-be-on-the-exam" case scenarios gives the examinee an obvious, clear-cut advantage. *Platinum Vignettes*™ were written to offer you that advantage.

You need to be familiar not only with pathophysiology, but also the work-up and management of several conditions to succeed on the USMLE Step 2 exam. Sifting through the history, physical exam findings, and various tests, you are expected to make and confirm the diagnosis and manage the patient's condition.

Each book in the *Platinum Vignettes*™ presents 50 case scenarios or clinical vignettes. The individual vignettes are followed by the diagnosis, pathophysiology, diagnostic strategies, and management issues pertaining to that specific patient. The reader must turn the page to obtain these latter details, and is encouraged to "guess" before reading about the patient's condition and course. In fact, you are advised not only to guess the diagnosis, but also to postulate on which test to order next, what therapy to give, and what to "watch out" for in the condition presented.

Important words or phrases ("buzzwords") are set in bold type in the explanation of each vignette. These words or phrases indicate the material most commonly asked about on the exam or are important in helping to distinguish one condition from another. This format is designed for review of material that was previously learned during rotations; therefore, further reading is advised if the topic or buzzwords are unfamiliar. Remember, buzzwords are rarely helpful unless you know what they mean!

Every attempt was made to provide the most current, up-to-date information on every topic tackled in this volume and every volume in the series—but medicine is a rapidly changing field. If you hear about a new therapy in a conference or on rounds, it may well be that the standard of care has changed. Remember, though, that what you see on the wards and in the office isn't always applicable to the boards (e.g., everyone with pneumonia should not be given the latest "big-gun" antibiotic; all patients with headaches should not receive a CT scan).

Good luck!

ADAM BROCHERT, MD

NOTE: A standard Table of Contents, with cases listed by diagnosis, would give you too much of a head start on solving each patient scenario. Challenge yourself! When ready, you can turn to the detailed Case Index at the back of this book.

Case 1

Internal Medicine

History

A 57-year-old man comes into the office complaining of fever and a cough. The man says he felt completely healthy 4 days ago, but on the following day started feeling feverish and coughed up yellowish-green phlegm the next morning. His symptoms have progressively worsened. He also mentions that his chest hurts on the right side when he takes a deep breath. The patient says his wife was sick with milder but similar symptoms a week or two ago.

The patient's past medical history includes hypertension and arthritis. His medications include metoprolol and celecoxib. He smokes roughly a pack of cigarettes per day, but does not drink alcohol or use other drugs.

Exam

T: 102.4°F BP: 128/86 RR: 18/min. P: 94/min.

The patient appears mildly tachypneic, but is not in distress. Head and neck exams are unremarkable. Chest exam reveals decreased breath sounds in the upper right lung field, with dullness to percussion as well as egophony and increased tactile fremitus in this area. The remaining lung fields are clear to auscultation. Cardiac, abdominal, and extremity exams are unremarkable.

Tests

Hemoglobin: 16 g/dL (normal 14–18)
White blood cell count: 14,900/μL (normal 4500–11,000)
Neutrophils: 87%
Platelets: 310,000/μL (normal 150,000–400,000)
Sodium: 137 meq/L (normal 135–145)
Potassium: 4.1 meq/L (normal 3.5–5)
BUN: 15 mg/dL (normal 8–25)
Creatinine: 1 mg/dL (normal 0.6–1.5)
AST: 17 u/L (normal 7–27)
Chest x-ray: see figure

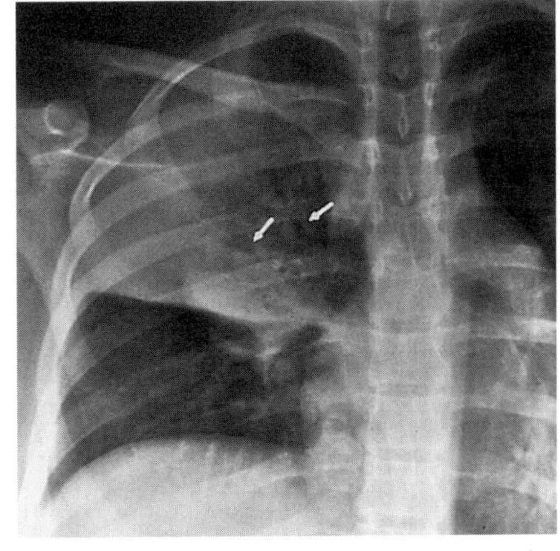

From Groskin SA: General principles and pattern recognition. In Katz DS, Math KR, Groskin SA (eds): Radiology Secrets. Philadelphia, Hanley & Belfus, Inc., 1998, pp 33–39; with permission.

Condition Typical community-acquired pneumonia

The chest x-ray reveals a lobar consolidation pattern in the right upper lobe with **air bronchograms** (*arrows*). The inferior margin of the pneumonia is the minor fissure.

Pathophysiology

Community-acquired pneumonia generally is considered either **typical** or **atypical**. Typical cases are usually due to ***Streptococcus pneumoniae,*** have less than 2 days of prodrome (e.g., headache, malaise), produce fever > 102°F, affect those over age 40, and involve a distinct lobe on chest x-ray. Atypical cases are due to one of several organisms (e.g., ***Mycoplasma, Chlamydia***) have more than 3 days of prodrome, fever < 102°F, affect those under age 40, and have diffuse or multilobe involvement on chest x-ray. The distinction is not always clear-cut clinically, however. Pneumonia is an extremely common infection and is roughly the **sixth leading cause of death** in the U.S.

Diagnosis & Treatment

Patients present with **fever, cough,** and **constitutional** symptoms (e.g., headache, malaise, arthralgias). **Pleuritic chest pain** may be present from irritation of the pleura. **Tachypnea** is common. Severe cases can present with septic shock (signs such as severe **hypoxia, tachycardia, hypotension,** warm and **flushed skin, oliguria** and/or altered mental status are present in this setting). Patients may have recent **sick contacts. Smokers** and those at the **extremes of age** are at a higher risk, and it is not uncommon for pneumonia to develop after a viral upper respiratory infection, classically in the winter (flu season).

Physical exam often reveals signs of lobar consolidation with typical pneumonia. These include a fairly **focal area** of *decreased* breath sounds, **dullness** to percussion, and *increased* tactile fremitus. "**Bronchial**" breath sounds, **egophony** (patients say "e," you hear "a"), and **whispered pectoriloquy**/bronchophony (when patient whispers/talks, you hear it louder than usual) may all be heard when listening with a stethoscope. **Leukocytosis** with increased neutrophils is usually present. **Chest x-ray** confirms the diagnosis and classically reveals consolidation confined to one lobe. An **effusion** (parapneumonic) may be present as well.

Antibiotic treatment to cover commonly occurring organisms is given after sputum and blood cultures are drawn. **Azithromycin** or levofloxacin are appropriate to cover typical and atypical bugs while waiting for culture results.

More High-Yield Facts

Patients > **65 years old** or with **multiple medical problems** should be treated on an inpatient basis even if symptoms are mild, due to **increased mortality**.

Don't forget the pneumococcal and influenza **vaccines** as prevention.

Case 2

Internal Medicine

History

A 48-year-old woman is experiencing muscle weakness. She says the symptoms started about 7 days ago and have become progressively worse. She denies weight loss, fever, and other symptoms of infection. Past medical history includes hypertension and mild renal insufficiency. The patient takes propranolol for her hypertension. Captopril was also added to her hypertension regimen 10 days ago to improve blood pressure control. She also takes aspirin as needed for osteoarthritis; intake has been around-the-clock for the past week due to a "flare" of her symptoms.

Exam

T: 98.5°F BP: 148/90 RR: 16/min. P: 84/min.

The patient is no acute distress. Head, neck, chest, and abdominal exams are unremarkable. Rectal exam reveals no masses and stool that is negative for occult blood. Extremity exam demonstrates symmetric, mild muscle weakness in both arms and legs, with no focal deficit identified. Reflexes are normal.

Tests

Hemoglobin: 14 mg/dL (normal 12–16)
White blood cell count: 6800/μL (normal 4500–11,000)
Platelets: 270,000/μL (normal 150,000–400,000)
Basic chemistry panel: pending
EKG: see figure

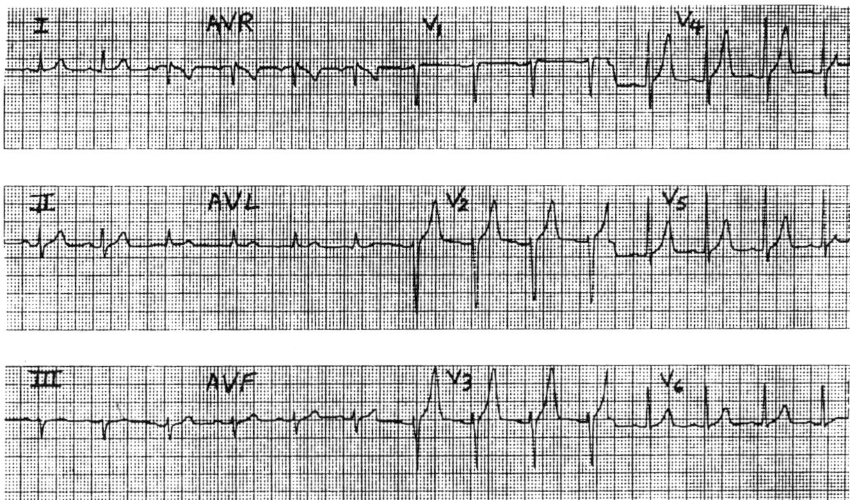

From Seelig CB: Simplified EKG Analysis. Philadelphia, Hanley & Belfus, Inc., 1992, pp 107–110; with permission.

Condition

Hyperkalemia

The EKG shows the classic, tall, peaked, "tented" T waves (most prominent in leads V2–V5).

Pathophysiology

Hyperkalemia is mainly clinically significant for its **cardiac effects,** which can be lethal. Causes include **renal failure** or dysfunction (e.g., renal tubular acidosis), **medications** (**NSAIDs, aspirin, ACE-Inhibitors,** potassium-sparing diuretics such as **spironolactone** and **beta-blockers**), severe **tissue destruction** (muscle necrosis, burns), **hypoaldosteronism, acidosis,** and **adrenal insufficiency**.

Diagnosis & Treatment

Hyperkalemia is often **asymptomatic** until cardiac effects occur, but can cause **muscle weakness**. The diagnosis is made from an **elevated serum potassium level** or typical **EKG** findings. **Peaked T waves** occur first, progressing to widening of the QRS, prolonged PR interval, loss of P waves, and a sine wave pattern. **Asystole** or **ventricular fibrillation** can occur with severe toxicity.

Treatment involves first *stopping* any aggravating medications (this patient's hyperkalemia is from the combination of ACE-inhibitor, aspirin, and propranolol). Most patients are then treated with **oral sodium polystyrene** resin. If the potassium level is > **6.5** or cardiac toxicity is apparent (more than just peaked T waves), **prompt intravenous therapy** is generally given. **Calcium gluconate** is given first for its cardioprotective effects, even though it doesn't affect the serum potassium level. Next, **sodium bicarbonate** can be given to cause alkalosis and drive potassium intracellularly. **Insulin** (given with glucose to prevent hypoglycemia) is also used for this "cellular shift" effect. Oral treatment can be given at the same time to effect lowering of the total body potassium load. If these treatments fail, **dialysis** is generally needed.

More High-Yield Facts

If the potassium is high, but the patient is totally asymptomatic and has a normal EKG, the likely cause is **hemolysis** of the lab specimen and **false** ("spurious") hyperkalemia. **Repeat the test** and/or ask the lab about hemolysis.

Hyporeninemic hypoaldosteronism (type **IV** renal tubular acidosis) is a classic cause of hyperkalemia in patients with diabetes. Those with **diabetic ketoacidosis** may present with hyperkalemia, but the overall body potassium is low, and the high potassium is due to acidosis and insulin deficiency. Treating the ketoacidosis will normalize the potassium *without* the need for specific hyperkalemia therapy.

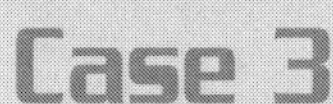

Case 3

Internal Medicine

History

A 39-year-old man presents with muscle weakness and skin discoloration. He says that both came on gradually over the last few weeks. He also mentions excessive weight gain, easy bruising, and irritability. His past medical history is unremarkable, and he takes no regular medications. The patient last saw a doctor 8 months ago and was given a "clean bill of health." He does not smoke, drink alcohol, or use illicit drugs. Family history is notable for heart disease.

Exam

T: 98.8°F   BP: 168/94   RR: 16/min.   P: 80/min.

The patient is no acute distress, but has fairly marked truncal obesity. No scleral icterus or ocular abnormalities are noted. His chest is clear to auscultation, and there are no heart murmurs. Abdominal exam reveals an unusual appearance of the abdominal wall skin (see figure). Bowel sounds are normal; no masses are palpable. Extremity exam reveals some mild wasting symmetrically. Muscle strength is 5/5 in both upper and lower extremities, with 4/5 strength noted in the hip flexors bilaterally. No side-to-side asymmetry is noted, and reflexes are normal.

Tests

Hemoglobin: 17 mg/dL (normal 14–18)
White blood cell count: 6000/μL (normal 4500–11,000)
Platelets: 270,000/μL (normal 150,000–400,000)
Sodium: 148 meq/L (normal 135–145)
Potassium: 3.1 meq/L (normal 3.5–5)
BUN: 20 mg/dL (normal 8–25)
Creatinine: 1.1 mg/dL (normal 0.6–1.5)
Glucose, fasting: 150 mg/dL (normal fasting 70–110)

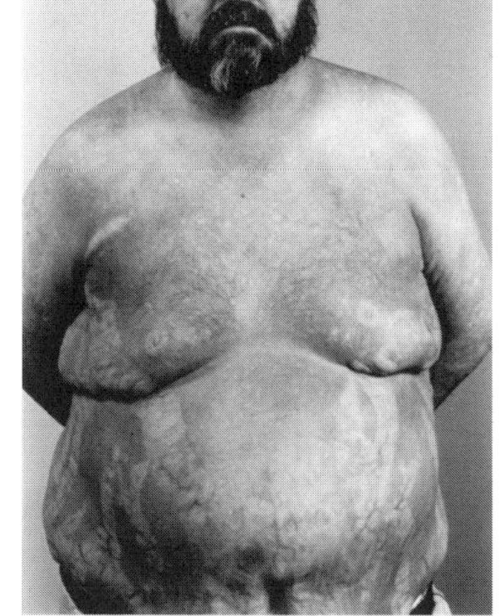

From Fitzpatrick JE, Aeling JL (eds): Dermatology Secrets. Philadelphia, Hanley & Belfus, Inc., 1996, pp 241–246; with permission.

Condition Cushing syndrome

The photo reveals truncal obesity and abdominal striae, which are classic.

Pathophysiology

Cushing syndrome is due to glucocorticoid hormone excess. It is most commonly seen in those taking pharmacologic doses of corticosteroids. In those not taking steroids, 75% have an **ACTH-secreting pituitary microadenoma** (known as Cushing's *disease*). Other causes include other ACTH-secreting neoplasms (classic is **small cell lung cancer**), benign **adrenal adenomas,** and (rarely) **adrenal carcinoma** or primary adrenal hyperplasia.

Corticosteroid excess spares few organ systems; thus any decision to initiate prolonged steroid treatment must include a careful evaluation of the **risks and benefits** of therapy as well as **close monitoring** during therapy.

Diagnosis & Treatment

Classic symptoms include **truncal obesity** with extremity wasting, **"moon" facies** (round, reddened face)**, easy bruising, purplish skin striae,** acne, **hirsutism, amenorrhea/oligomenorrhea, muscle weakness** (from steroid myopathy, mostly affecting the proximal muscles), **irritability, psychiatric disturbances (depression, psychosis, emotional lability), insomnia,** and **memory problems**. A history of steroid use is obviously important.

Physical and lab findings include the above plus **hypertension, peripheral edema, hyperglycemia**/glucose intolerance, **osteoporosis,** and mild **hypernatremia** and **hypokalemia**. There is also increased risk of **infection**.

The diagnosis is confirmed with a **24-hour urinary free cortisol** measurement. A dexamethasone suppression test is a less desirable option. After the initial diagnosis is made, the cause for Cushing syndrome must be sought. An **ACTH level** can be measured: high ACTH means there is an ACTH-secreting neoplasm; low ACTH means there is a primary adrenal problem. Other lab tests can be performed, but are not likely to be asked about on Step 2. **MRI** can usually confirm a pituitary neoplasm, and **CT of the abdomen** can detect adrenal masses or enlargement. A small cell lung cancer is usually already diagnosed by the time it causes Cushing syndrome.

Treatment is **resection** of the neoplasm, **stopping/lowering** the steroid dose (if possible), treatment of lung cancer, etc. depending on the cause.

More High-Yield Facts

Aminoglutethimide or **metyrapone** can be used to inhibit steroid synthesis in those who are not surgical candidates. **Mitotane,** which destroys cortisol-secreting adrenal cells, is another option.

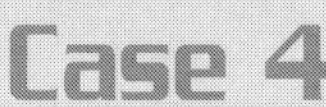

Case 4

Internal Medicine

History

A 39-year-old man seeks a routine check-up. He says he has not seen a doctor in 10 years and thought it was time he had a physical exam. He has no complaints. Past medical history is unremarkable, and the patient takes no regular medications. He is a construction worker who drinks 4–5 beers after work a few nights a week and smokes one-half pack of cigarettes per day. He denies the use of illicit drugs. Family history is notable for heart disease and hypertension (HTN).

Exam

T: 98.6°F   BP: 148/92   RR: 12/min.   P: 78/min.

The patient is overweight. The head and neck exam is unremarkable. His chest is clear to auscultation, and no heart murmurs are noted. Abdominal, rectal, extremity, and neurologic exams are normal.

Tests

Hemoglobin: 16 mg/dL (normal 14–18)
White blood cell count: 6700/μL (normal 4500–11,000)
Platelets: 270,000/μL (normal 150,000–400,000)
Sodium: 140 meq/L (normal 135–145)
Potassium: 4.1 meq/L (normal 3.5–5)
BUN: 10 mg/dL (normal 8–25)
Creatinine: 1 mg/dL (normal 0.6–1.5)
AST: 12 u/L (normal 7–27)
Glucose, fasting: 90 mg/dL (normal fasting 70–110)
Urinalysis: negative for glucose, protein, bacteria, white blood cells, and red blood cells. Normal specific gravity.

Condition Elevated blood pressure

Pathophysiology

Most (**90–95%**) cases of HTN are **essential** (idiopathic or primary). Other causes are called **secondary** and include **renal artery stenosis, endocrine abnormalities** (e.g., Cushing's, Conn's, pheochromocytoma), **renal insufficiency/failure,** and **coarctation of the aorta**. Other common causes of secondary HTN are **excess alcohol consumption** in males and **oral contraceptive** use in females.

Diagnosis & Treatment

HTN is **asymptomatic**. Rare exceptions are hypertensive emergencies and symptoms from secondary causes of HTN. The diagnosis is made by measuring a **systolic blood pressure ≥ 140 mmHg** or a **diastolic blood pressure ≥ 90 mmHg** on **three separate occasions**. Exceptions to the three-measurement rule are hypertensive emergencies and new-onset HTN in pregnancy.

Initial labs include a **complete blood count, urinalysis,** and **basic chemistry** panel, which help detect most secondary causes (along with the history). An **EKG** is also usually performed to check for effects of HTN on the heart (e.g., left ventricular hypertrophy). Treatment starts with **lifestyle modification** in cases of essential HTN. This involves 3–6 months of healthy **diet** (low salt, cholesterol, and calories), **exercise, weight reduction,** and **decreased smoking and alcohol** intake (oral contraceptive pills should also be stopped). If these measures fail, medications are employed. The four first-line agents for HTN are **beta blockers, thiazide diuretics, ACE-inhibitors,** and **calcium-channel blockers**.

More High-Yield Facts

Lowering blood pressure in those with HTN lowers the risk for **stroke** (most important risk factor), **coronary artery disease/atherosclerosis, myocardial infarction, renal failure,** and **dissecting aortic aneurysms. Heart disease** is the number one cause of death in patients with untreated HTN (as in the general population).

Isolated systolic or diastolic HTN **should be treated** if it persists. The elderly are prone to systolic HTN, due to decreased vascular compliance.

HTN **screening** is needed roughly every 2 years for life (start at age 3).

Standard HTN agents are poor choices during pregnancy (though labetalol has gained acceptance). Counsel/choose appropriately when treating **reproductive-age females,** who may become pregnant during therapy.

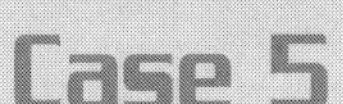

Case 5

Internal Medicine

History

A 58-year-old man has come to the emergency department because of severe shortness of breath and nausea. He says the symptoms started suddenly an hour ago when he became angry at work. He experiences similar, milder forms of these symptoms whenever he exerts himself, but they disappear once he has rested, and he has never told anyone about these episodes. Past medical history is significant for diabetes and hypertension, both for more than 15 years. The patient was also told previously that his cholesterol was high, but he refused to take medications for the problem. He takes enalapril and glipizide. The patient has smoked two packs of cigarettes per day for the past 25 years, but drinks alcohol only rarely. Family history is notable for heart attacks in the patient's father and one of his brothers.

Exam

T: 98.9°F BP: 158/92 RR: 22/min. P: 102/min.

The patient is anxious, diaphoretic, and tachypneic. He also appears pale. His chest is clear to auscultation. Cardiac exam reveals no murmurs. Abdominal, rectal, extremity, and neurologic exams are unremarkable.

Tests

Hemoglobin: 17 mg/dL (normal 14–18) WBCs: 9900/μL
Sodium: 140 meq/L (normal 135–145) Potassium: 4.1 meq/L (normal 3.5–5)
Creatinine: 1.2 mg/dL (normal 0.6–1.5) EKG: see figure
Urinalysis: negative for glucose, protein, bacteria, white blood cells, and red blood cells; normal specific gravity

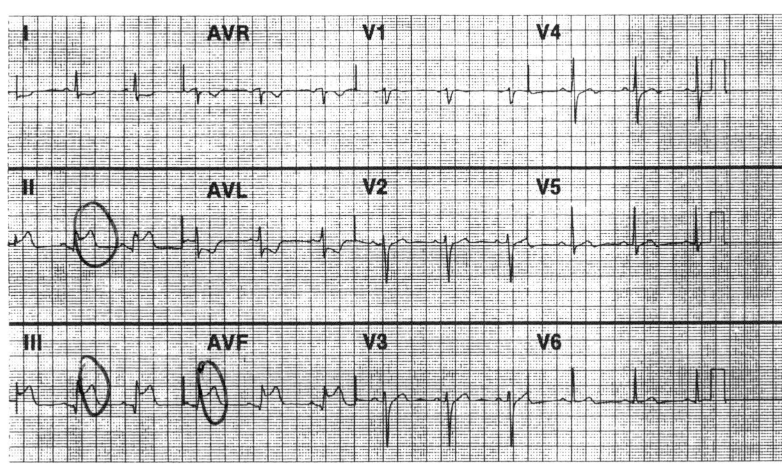

From Habib GB, Zollo Jr AJ: Cardiology. Zollo Jr AJ (ed): Medical Secrets, 2nd ed. Philadelphia, Hanley & Belfus, Inc., 1997, pp 59–95; with permission.

Condition

Myocardial infarction (MI)

The EKG shows marked ST elevation and early Q wave formation in **leads II, III, and aVF** (the inferior leads), indicating an **inferior wall** infarct.

Pathophysiology

Most cases of MI are due to the long-standing effects of **atherosclerosis** of the coronary arteries. Risk factors for coronary artery disease (CAD) include **age** ($\geq$ 45 for men, $\geq$ 55 for women), **family history** (MI or sudden death in first-degree male relative < 55 years old or female relative < 65), **current cigarette smoking, hypertension, diabetes mellitus,** and **hypercholesterolemia** or **low HDL** cholesterol ($\leq$ 35 mg/dL). Other risk factors are more controversial and include "**type A**" personality, **obesity,** sedentary lifestyle, homocysteine, chlamydial infection, and stress.

Diagnosis & Treatment

Classic symptoms of an MI include **chest pain** (substernal, crushing or pressure-like pain that may radiate to the jaw and/or left shoulder/arm), **shortness of breath, sweating, nausea/vomiting,** and/or anxiety. Twenty percent of patients (one-third of **diabetic** patients) have a **"silent" MI** (i.e., no chest pain).

Physical findings may include the above plus t**achycardia, tachypnea,** and **pallor**. A new **heart murmur** or **arrhythmia** may be present. Signs of congestive heart failure or shock may be present with larger heart attacks.

The diagnosis is confirmed using the **EKG** (ST segment elevation and/or Q waves are classic), which is abnormal in a **specific** heart **segment** (e.g., inferior or anterior leads), and **cardiac enzyme** levels. Commonly used enzymes are **CPK/CK-MB** (CPK is nonspecific, CK-MB is specific for myocardium; both should be elevated in an MI) and **troponin I or P**. These are measured every 8 hours for 24 hours before MI is ruled out. Lactate dehydrogenase (**LDH "flip"** or $LDH_1 > LDH_2$) or troponins are useful after 24 hours (CPK level may return to normal by this time).

Basic treatment includes **aspirin** and a **beta-blocker** (both clearly improve survival), as well as **oxygen, nitrates/morphine** for pain relief, and EKG monitoring (give **lidocaine** if sustained ventricular tachycardia develops). **Thrombolysis** and/or **angioplasty** are options in those who present **within 4–6 hours. HMG-CoA reductase inhibitors** have recently been shown to reduce mortality in the acute setting. **ACE-inhibitors** reduce mortality acutely in those who develop heart failure from the MI.

More High-Yield Facts

If an MI occurs in a **pediatric** patient, think of **Kawasaki syndrome**.

Case 6

Internal Medicine

History

A 28-year-old man complains of "spots" on his eyelids and his feet. He says they have been present for several years, but he now wants to investigate having them removed. He has no other symptoms and hasn't seen a doctor in 10 years. Past medical history is unremarkable, and the patient takes no medications. He is a vegetarian and does not smoke or drink alcohol. Family history is notable for high cholesterol levels and heart attacks at an early age in several first- and second-degree relatives.

Exam

T: 98.5°F BP: 118/76 RR: 12/min. P: 72/min.

The patient appears healthy and in no acute distress. In addition to the eyelid lesions (see figure), there are large, palpable, similarly colored nodules attached to the Achilles tendons bilaterally. The chest, abdominal, and neurologic exams are unremarkable.

Tests

Hemoglobin: 16 mg/dL (normal 14–18)
White blood cell count: 7900/μL (normal 4500–11,000)
Platelets: 250,000/μL (normal 150,000–400,000)
EKG: normal

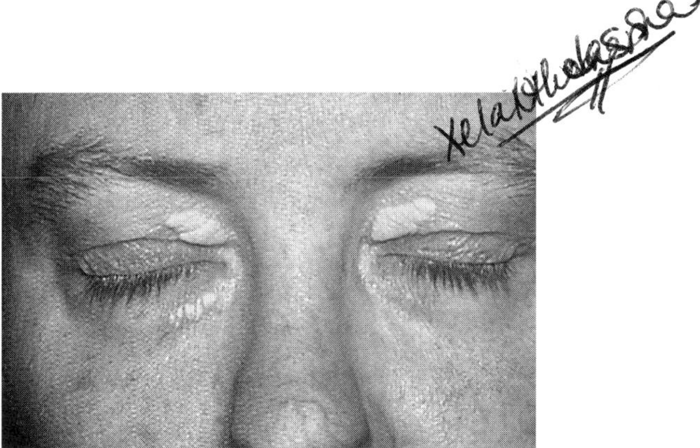

From Gault JA: Eyelid tumors. In Vander JF, Gault JA (eds): Ophthalmology Secrets. Philadelphia, Hanley & Belfus, Inc., 1998, pp 252–256; with permission.

Condition Familial hyperlipidemia (primary hyperlipoproteinemia)

The photo reveals xanthelasma, which can be a marker for this condition.

Pathophysiology

There are several types of FH, which can affect chylomicron, triglyceride, very-low-density lipoprotein (VLDL), and/or low-density lipoprotein (LDL) levels. The types that elevate LDL and/or VLDL (primarily familial hypercholesterolemia or type 2) increase the risk of **atherosclerosis** and **coronary artery disease**. The types that elevate triglycerides/chylomicrons (primarily type 1) classically cause **pancreatitis**.

Diagnosis & Treatment

The diagnosis of familial high cholesterol is suggested in those with a **strong family history** who present with **xanthelasma** (which can be a normal finding in healthy adults or a sign of high cholesterol) or **tuberous xanthomas** (Achilles tendon lesions or lesions on the palms are classic). **Eruptive xanthomas** (small papules on the buttocks, thighs, or elbows) or idiopathic and/or recurrent **pancreatitis** are markers for familial cases that cause high triglyceride levels. Patients may be completely **asymptomatic**.

Any of the above presentations should prompt evaluation of the patient's lipid levels. A **fasting lipoprotein analysis** measures **total cholesterol, high-density lipoprotein** (HDL), and **triglyceride** levels. **LDL** levels can be determined directly or **calculated** using the formula

LDL = total cholesterol–HDL–(triglycerides/5).

Treatment involves **diet modifications** (often less effective in this setting, but a low-fat diet is important), alteration of any other coronary artery disease **risk factors** (e.g., quit smoking, control blood pressure), and **medications**. Treatment of elevated cholesterol includes **niacin, bile acid sequestrants** (e.g., **cholestyramine**), and **HMG-CoA reductase inhibitors** (e.g., simvastatin, lovastatin). For elevated triglycerides, use **gemfibrozil** or **nicotinic acid** (a less desirable second-line agent is clofibrate).

More High-Yield Facts

Test all **family members,** even if asymptomatic, when an index case of familial hyperlipidemia is found.

Xanthelasma can be a **normal finding** in those with normal cholesterol levels, but on the boards it is more likely to represent high cholesterol. Check a fasting lipid panel in any patient with xanthelasma. Xanthelasma can be removed (using a laser) if desired for cosmetic reasons.

Familial hypercholesterolemia is **common** (affects 1 in 500 persons) and is **autosomal dominant**. Cholesterol/LDL is elevated and triglycerides are normal in this condition.

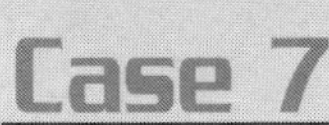

Internal Medicine

History

A 27-year-old woman is suffering from alternating constipation and diarrhea, as well as occasional abdominal bloating. These symptoms have been going on for several months. Her abdominal pain is generally relieved after she has a bowel movement. She says her stools often appear to contain mucus and are typically loose and pebble-shaped when she is not constipated. The patient denies fever, weight loss, hematochezia, melena, and sick contacts. She is an office manager with a high level of stress at work.

Past medical history is unremarkable, though the patient does admit to occasional bouts of depression. She takes no medications, other than acetaminophen as needed for abdominal pain. The patient does not smoke, drink alcohol, or use illicit drugs. She rarely drinks milk or uses dairy products. There is no family history of bowel problems.

Exam

T: 98.5°F BP: 116/74 RR: 14/min. P: 66/min.

The patient appears healthy and in no acute distress. Head, neck, and chest exams are unremarkable. Abdominal exam reveals normal bowel sounds and no abdominal distension. The patient is not tender to palpation, and no masses are appreciated. No masses are found on rectal exam, and mucus-containing stool is negative for occult blood. The pelvic exam is normal. The rest of the examination is unremarkable.

A sigmoidoscopy reveals no abnormalities.

Tests

Hemoglobin: 14 mg/dL (normal 12–16)
White blood cell count: 7200/μL (normal 4500–11,000)
Platelets: 250,000/μL (normal 150,000–400,000)
Stool: negative for pathologic bacteria, ova, and parasites; no white or red blood cells
Ultrasound of the abdomen: no abnormalities

Irritable bowel syndrome (IBS)

Pathophysiology

IBS is characterized by the presence of **altered bowel habits** and **abdominal discomfort** in the **absence of detectable organic pathology**. Symptoms are generally **chronic**. This disorder is **common** and usually begins **before the age of 30,** with **females** affected more commonly than males. IBS is thought to account for up to one-third of all outpatient gastroenterology visits. The disorder is considered "**functional,**" as no cause has been identified. Those with psychiatric/emotional disorders or a history of psychological or sexual abuse are more likely to be affected.

Diagnosis & Treatment

Classic symptoms include **abdominal pain** (classically **relieved by defecation**), an **altered frequency** of bowel movements (**alternating** diarrhea and constipation is classic), an **altered consistency** of stool (**mucus-containing stools are classic,** as are **pebble-like stools** and **loose stools**), a **sensation of incomplete evacuation,** and a sensation of **bloating** or **abdominal distension**. This history alone, if present for **at least 3 months,** is virtually diagnostic of IBS. Patients often report a history of **stress** (which can aggravate symptoms) and may mention **psychiatric/emotional disturbances**.

Physical findings are generally *absent,* though abdominal discomfort may be present with palpation. Any tests done are *negative* for pathology. In all patients with IBS, a **sigmoidoscopy or barium enema** to rule out inflammatory bowel disease, malignancy, and diverticulosis as well as a test of the **stool** for **giardiasis** or other enteric pathogens are usually done. Also consider **lactase deficiency,** as this is a common problem (removal of dairy products from the diet makes symptoms go away).

Treatment includes **reassurance/support, stress reduction, dietary measures** (**increased fiber** is always prescribed, avoidance of exacerbating foods), and possibly **adjunctive medications** to treat specific symptoms (antispasmodics, antidiarrheals, laxatives, antidepressants, anxiolytics). **Psychiatric referral** may be indicated in some patients.

More High-Yield Facts

In a **child** with vague abdominal complaints and a negative work-up, consider **separation anxiety** or **child abuse. Abused adult women** may also present with vague abdominal complaints.

Patients with weight loss, fever, anemia, or other signs do *not* have irritable bowel syndrome, and another cause for their symptoms should be sought.

Case 8

Internal Medicine

History

A 32-year-old woman complains of nervousness, fatigue, palpitations, irritability, and "feeling hot all the time." She has also noticed that her eyes "look funny," and the skin over her shins has a rash on it. She says her symptoms have come on gradually over the last few months and continue to get worse. Further questioning reveals weight loss, trouble sleeping, and amenorrhea for the past 10 weeks, though the patient's menstrual cycles are usually quite regular. The patient's past medical history is unremarkable, and she takes no medications. She is not sexually active and does not smoke or use alcohol.

Exam

T: 99.1°F BP: 130/86 RR: 16/min.
P: 70–120/min. (varies)

The patient appears anxious and is restless and fidgety. Her skin is warm and moist. Her eyes do have an unusual appearance (see figure, *top*). A rash is present on her shins (see figure, *bottom*). Neck exam reveals symmetric thyroid enlargement, with no discrete masses palpable. Her lungs are clear to auscultation. Cardiac exam reveals an irregularly irregular rhythm; no murmurs are appreciated. Abdominal, pelvic, and rectal exams are unremarkable. You notice a fine tremor in her hands when the patient tries to hold her arms outstretched and still.

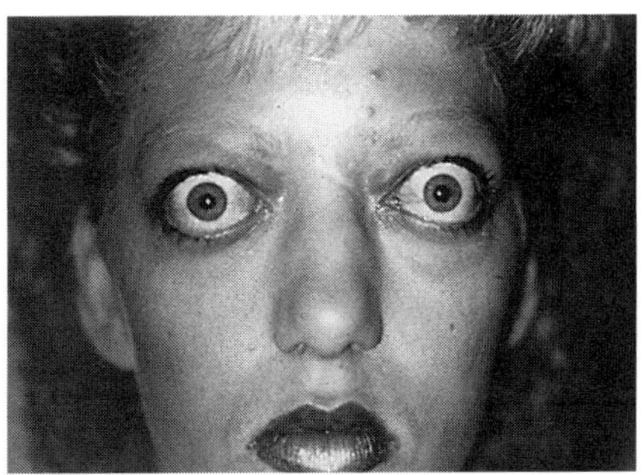

From Penne RB. In Vander JF, Gault JA (eds): Ophthalmology Secrets. Philadelphia, Hanley & Belfus, Inc., 1998, pp 239–243; with permission

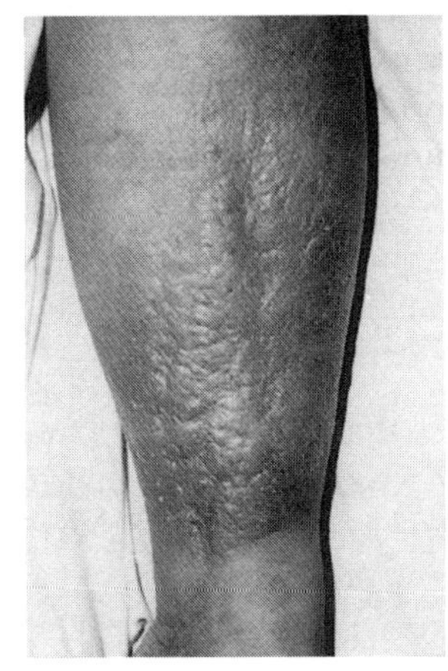

From Fitzpatrick JE. In McDermott MT (ed): Endocrine Secrets, 3rd ed. Philadelphia, Hanley & Belfus, Inc., 2002, pp 421–428; with permission.

Tests

Hemoglobin: 12 mg/dL (normal 12–16)
White blood cell count: 7500/μL (normal 4500–11,000)
Platelets: 330,000/μL (normal 150,000–400,000)
Urinalysis: negative for glucose, protein, bacteria, and white blood cells
B-HCG, qualitative: negative

Condition Graves' disease

The top photo shows proptosis and lid retraction from Graves' ophthalmopathy, and the bottom photo demonstrates pretibial myxedema.

Pathophysiology

Graves' disease is due to **thyroid-stimulating immunoglobulins / antibodies,** which generally cause hyperthyroidism. Thus, the gland functions outside the control of the hypothalamic/pituitary axis. Graves' usually occurs in **reproductive-age females** (outnumber men by 5–10:1).

Other causes of hyperthyroidism include **toxic adenoma, toxic multinodular goiter** (Plummer's disease), excess consumption of thyroid hormone (either iatrogenic or due to **factitious disorder**), and **subacute thyroiditis** (the thyroid gland is classically tender, thought to be caused by a viral infection). Exotic causes include a TSH-secreting pituitary adenoma, thyroid carcinoma, amiodarone, and struma ovarii (an ovarian teratoma).

Diagnosis & Treatment

Symptoms of hyperthyroidism include **anxiety/nervousness, irritability, emotional lability, insomnia, heat intolerance, sweating, palpitations, tremors, weight loss** (usually with **increased appetite**), **fatigue, weakness, diarrhea,** and **oligo- or amenorrhea**.

Physical exam findings may include the above plus an **enlarged thyroid gland** (goiter, which may be symmetric [Graves'] or asymmetric [toxic nodule/toxic multinodular goiter]); **tachycardia; atrial fibrillation** (irregularly irregular heartbeat); warm, moist skin; and fine, silky hair. **Eye findings** (proptosis, lid lag, infrequent blinking) and **pretibial myxedema** are *specific* for Graves' disease (not seen with other causes). In Graves' disease, the **TSH level is low** (may be undetectable), and the **T3 and T4 levels are high**. The diagnosis of Graves' and toxic nodule/goiter is often confirmed with a nuclear medicine thyroid scan (whole gland is "hot" in Graves'; only specific areas are "hot" with a nodule/goiter).

Treatment for Graves' disease includes **antithyroid drugs** (e.g., propylthiouracil, methimazole) and/or **beta-blockers,** but these are temporary measures. The definitive treatment is **radioactive iodine,** which **destroys** the thyroid gland (at least 40% of patients eventually become **hypothyroid** and will need hormone replacement; this is one of the **common causes** of hypothyroidism). **Surgical removal** of the gland is another option, but is often reserved for **pregnant** patients, in whom radioactive iodine is avoided (crosses the placenta).

More High-Yield Facts

If a patient presents with new-onset **atrial fibrillation,** check a **TSH level**.

Case 9

Internal Medicine

History

A 62-year-old black woman is experiencing fatigue, weakness, and tingling and numbness in both of her legs. All of her symptoms have come on gradually over the past few months. The patient's past medical history is remarkable only for "lightening" of her skin, which has been present for many years, and arthritis. Her only medication is occasional acetaminophen for arthritis. The patient does not smoke or drink alcohol and is sexually active only with her husband of 35 years.

Exam

T: 98.3°F BP: 126/84 RR: 18/min. P: 94/min.

The patient is mildly tachypneic, but in no acute distress. Her skin appears depigmented (see figure, *top*). Her sclera and mucous membranes are pale, and her tongue is smooth and "beefy" red. The lungs are clear to auscultation, and no cardiac murmurs are appreciated. Abdominal, pelvic, and rectal exams are unremarkable; stool is negative for occult blood. Extremity exam reveals a decreased vibratory sense in both lower extremities up to the knee and slightly impaired position sense. Reflexes are normal.

Tests

Hemoglobin: 9 mg/dL (normal 12–16)
White blood cell count: 4300/μL (normal 4500–11,000)
Platelets: 120,000/μL (normal 150,000–400,000)
Mean corpuscular volume (MCV): 114 μm/cell (normal 80–100)
Ferritin: 190 μg/dL (normal 20–200)
Peripheral blood smear: see figure, *bottom*

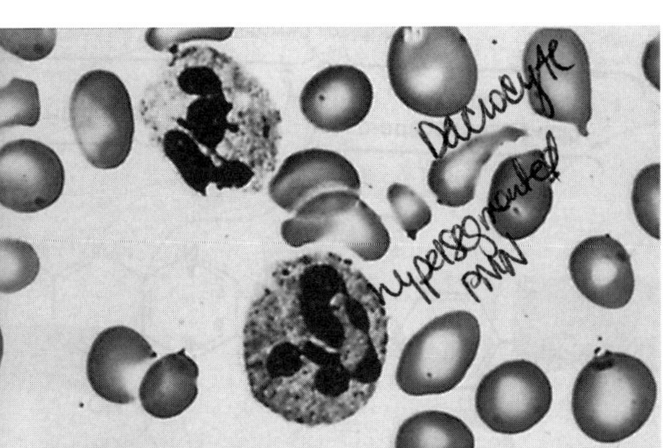

From Bonner H, Erslev AJ: The blood and lymphoid organs. In Rubin E, Farber JL (eds): Pathology, 2nd ed. Philadelphia, Lippincott, 1994, pp 994–1096; with permission.

Condition Pernicious anemia

The top photo depicts vitiligo, and the bottom photo shows hypersegmented neutrophils (classic!) and large oval erythrocytes with poikilocytosis (irregular shape of red blood cells).

Pathophysiology

Pernicious anemia is due to vitamin B_{12} deficiency from **antiparietal cell antibodies** that destroy intrinsic factor–secreting parietal cells. Without intrinsic factor, vitamin B_{12} cannot be absorbed, resulting in deficiency. This leads to megaloblastic anemia and neurological symptoms. Other **autoimmune disorders,** such as vitiligo, Graves' disease, hypothyroidism, and Addison's disease may coexist and point to pernicious anemia as the cause of B_{12} deficiency.

Other less common causes of B_{12} deficiency include **gastric or ileal resection,** small bowel **malabsorption** (e.g., celiac sprue, Crohn's disease), bacterial overgrowth (usually seen after bowel surgery), and, of course, *Diphyllobothrium latum* (fish tapeworm) infection.

Diagnosis & Treatment

Symptoms of vitamin B_{12} deficiency include those of **anemia** (fatigue, weakness, shortness of breath, palpitations) and **neurologic** symptoms (classic are **numbness and paresthesias in the lower extremities,** but **ataxia, irritability,** and **dementia** may also occur).

Physical findings include those of **anemia** (scleral and mucous membrane pallor) and **neurologic signs (decreased vibratory sense** is most common, though **decreased position sense, reflex changes,** and/or a positive **Romberg** test or **Babinski** sign may be present). A **smooth, beefy-red tongue** may also be seen. Blood tests reveal a **megaloblastic anemia** (MCV > 100), and the peripheral smear classically shows **hypersegmented neutrophils** (≥ 6 nuclear lobes), large red blood cells, and bizarre, misshapen platelets. **Leukopenia** and **thrombocytopenia** are also common. The vitamin B_{12} level is low, but this fact typically isn't given on the Step 2 exam.

The cause of B_{12} deficiency is determined with the **Schilling test**. This test involves giving oral **radioactive B_{12}** and measuring the radioactivity in the urine, which should be abnormally low due to malabsorption. The test is then repeated with the addition of oral intrinsic factor, which should normalize absorption if the cause is pernicious anemia. Treatment is vitamin B_{12} replacement for life, given via **monthly intramuscular injections**. Neurologic deficits may be *permanent*.

More High-Yield Facts

Folate and vitamin B_{12} deficiency both cause megaloblastic anemia, but only B_{12} deficiency causes neurologic symptoms.

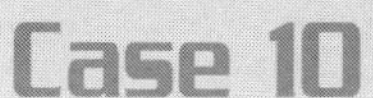

Internal Medicine

History

A 62-year-old postmenopausal woman visits your office for a check-up. She has not seen a doctor in 15 years and figures that she needs a “physical.” The patient saw a television show yesterday about screening for breast cancer and asks if she needs this or any other tests to look for cancer. She denies any symptoms and says she is healthy and active. Her past medical history is remarkable only for occasional heartburn, for which she takes occasional antacids. She does not smoke or drink alcohol, has been married for 40 years, and has three healthy children. She goes for 30-minute walks three times per week. Her family history is remarkable for heart disease and strokes.

Exam

T: 98.3°F BP: 136/84 RR: 14/min. P: 74/min.

The patient appears healthy and athletic. Her physical examination is completely within normal limits. What cancer screening tests, if any, would you advise? How about a man her age with no symptoms or findings?

Tests

Hemoglobin: 14 mg/dL (normal 12–16)
White blood cell count: 7300/μL (normal 4500–11,000)
Platelets: 240,000/μL (normal 150,000–400,000)
Urinalysis: negative for glucose, protein, bacteria, and white blood cells
EKG: normal

Cancer screening in asymptomatic adults

Pathophysiology

Cancer screening is a form of **secondary prevention**—early detection that allows early intervention to decrease the morbidity and mortality of a condition. Many cancers can be detected in the **asymptomatic** phase. Screening is recommended only if it is **cost-effective** and results in **improved patient outcomes** (e.g., reduced morbidity and mortality).

Diagnosis & Treatment

The most important cancer screening exams are for cervical, colorectal, and breast cancer. **Cervical cancer** screening involves the use of a **Pap smear every 1–3 years** starting at **age 20** (or sooner if the patient becomes sexually active before age 20). **Breast cancer** screening involves **annual mammography** starting at the age of **50,** and most recommend mammogram **every 1–2 years** from **40 to 50** years old. In addition, **self-breast exams** are advised **every month** from age **20,** and **physician breast exams every 3 years** from ages **20 to 40** and **annually** after age **40**.

Colon cancer screening includes **annual digital rectal exam** (starting at age **40**) and **annual occult blood testing of the stool** (starting at age **50**). In addition, **sigmoidoscopy** or barium enema is advised **every 3–5 years** starting at age **50**.

A **pelvic exam** is advised every 3 years in women ages 20 to 40, and annually in women over age 40, to detect pelvic malignancies. A physical exam to detect **thyroid, testicular, prostate, lymph node, oral, and skin cancer** is advised every 3 years in adults ages 20 to 40 and annually after age 40. All of the above recommendations are from the American Cancer Society, though other screening recommendations are available. You will not get any board questions wrong if you follow the ACS guidelines.

More High-Yield Facts

Prostate cancer screening is becoming more accepted, though there is still some controversy as to the survival benefit gained. Men should be offered **annual** prostate-specific antigen testing after age 50. **Digital rectal exam** for prostate cancer should be performed **annually** in men over age **50** (men already need annual exam after age 40 for colorectal cancer screening, so this prostate screening test is widely accepted).

Endometrial biopsy at menopause to detect endometrial cancer is *controversial* and not generally recommended. **Do not screen for lung cancer** even in high-risk patients (no benefit shown, though trials using high-resolution CT scans are currently underway).

Case 11

Internal Medicine

History

A 34-year-old woman is experiencing repeated episodes of tingling and occasional numbness in her lips and tongue, as well as her feet. She says her symptoms started about 2 weeks ago and have been getting worse. The patient also mentions feeling depressed and irritable and has generalized muscle aches and cramps. Past medical history is notable only for Graves' disease, for which the patient had a total thyroidectomy 2 weeks ago. She denies pain or swelling at the surgical site. She takes no medications and does not smoke. Family history is noncontributory.

Exam

T: 98.6°F   P: 126/82   RR: 14/min.   P: 76/min.

The patient appears healthy and in no acute distress, though she does require you to repeat several of your questions due to apparent difficulty in paying attention. When you tap on the patient's face just anterior to the external auditory meatus, several of her muscles of facial expression on that side twitch. Neck exam reveals a clean, dry, and intact recent surgical scar. No neck masses are palpable. Chest is clear to auscultation, and no cardiac murmurs are appreciated. The abdominal, rectal, pelvic, and extremity exams are unremarkable.

You instruct the patient to hyperventilate, and after several seconds her paresthesias become pronounced and both her hands begin to have painful muscular spasms.

Tests

Hemoglobin: 14 mg/dL (normal 12–16)
White blood cell count: 7300/μL (normal 4500–11,000)
Platelets: 240,000/μL (normal 150,000–400,000)
Urinalysis: negative for glucose, protein, bacteria, and white blood cells
EKG: see figure

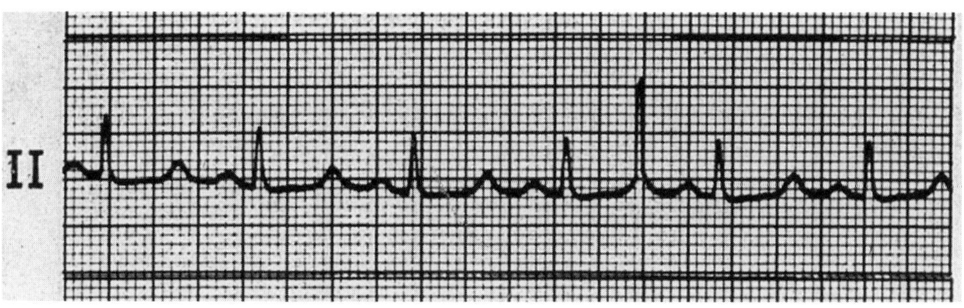

From Chung EK: Principles of Cardiac Arrhythmias, 4th ed. Phladelphia, Williams & Wilkins, 1989, pp 638–661; with permission.

Condition Hypocalcemia

The EKG shows marked **QT interval prolongation,** a classic finding in hypocalcemia.

Pathophysiology

The physiology of calcium is closely intertwined with that of **vitamin D, parathyroid hormone (PTH), phosphorus,** and **magnesium**. Hypocalcemia has several causes, including **post-thyroidectomy** if all four parathyroids are accidentally removed and/or damaged, **pseudohypoparathyroidism** (end-organ unresponsiveness to PTH), **DiGeorge's syndrome, vitamin D deficiency, renal failure/disease** (from deficient vitamin D formation and hyperphosphatemia), **hypomagnesemia, hypokalemia,** and **acute pancreatitis**. **Alkalosis** can temporarily cause or aggravate (as in this patient) hypocalcemia due to cellular shift.

Diagnosis & Treatment

The classic symptoms of hypocalcemia are **neurologic** and are known as **tetany,** which includes **paresthesias** (classically involving the **lips, tongue,** and **distal extremities**), **hand/foot/facial muscle spasms,** and **generalized muscle aches**. In addition, **irritability, depression,** and even psychosis, delirium, or dementia may occur.

Findings include **Chvostek's sign** (tapping on the facial nerve causes facial muscle contractions), **Trousseau's sign** (inflating a blood pressure cuff for 2–3 minutes causes hand muscle spasms), and **altered mental status**. The serum calcium and free (ionized) calcium levels are low. In the rare case when the cause is not clear, a **PTH level** can be checked to see if the problem is in the parathyroid glands (low PTH) or elsewhere (high PTH).

Treatment is directed at the cause. Most patients respond to **oral calcium** and **vitamin D** (e.g., cases due to hypoparathyroidism or renal failure).

More High-Yield Facts

The calcium and **albumin** levels are **closely related,** as albumin binds most of the serum calcium (inactive or nonionized calcium) and only a small percentage is unbound (active or ionized calcium). If the serum calcium level is low, **first check the albumin level** (or directly measure the ionized calcium level) to determine the significance. If the calcium and albumin levels are **both low,** the patient will be asymptomatic, and **treatment of the calcium level is not indicated,** as the ionized calcium level is normal.

Hypocalcemia is tough to correct if **hypomagnesemia** or **hypokalemia** are present. Check both these electrolytes in the setting of hypocalcemia and replace them at the same time as calcium if either is low.

Tetany in the first 48 hours of life = probable **DiGeorge's syndrome**.

Case 12

Internal Medicine

History

A 44-year-old recent immigrant from Haiti presents to the emergency department complaining of cough and malaise. His symptoms came on gradually over the past several months, but have gotten worse. The cough is "deep," according to the patient, and minimally productive of whitish sputum that is occasionally streaked with blood. He also mentions fever and profuse sweating at night, and thinks he has lost weight over the past few months. He denies any history of recent sick contacts. Past medical history is unremarkable, and the patient takes no medications. He does smoke and drink alcohol occasionally and mentions that he spent a few years in prison before coming to the United States.

Exam

T: 100.8°F BP: 124/80 RR: 16/min. P: 80/min.

The patient appears unkempt, somewhat cachectic, and chronically ill, though he is in no acute distress. Scleral pallor is noted, but the head and neck exams are otherwise unremarkable. There are rales in both upper lung fields, right greater than left. The remaining lung fields are clear. No cardiac murmurs are appreciated. The rest of the physical examination is unremarkable.

Tests

Hemoglobin: 11 mg/dL (normal 14–18)
Mean corpuscular volume: 85 μm/cell (normal 80–100)
White blood cell count: 7300/μL (normal 4500–11,000)
Platelets: 240,000/μL (normal 150,000–400,000)
Ferritin: 260 μg/L (normal 20–200)
Sodium: 133 meq/L (normal 135–145)
Potassium: 4.1 meq/L (normal 3.5–5)
BUN: 10 mg/dL (normal 8–25)
Creatinine: 0.9 mg/dL (normal 0.6–1.5)
Chest x-ray: see figure

From Hoeprich PD, Jordan MC (eds): Infectious Diseases, 4th ed. Philadelphia, Lippincott, 1989, pp 405–435; with permission.

Condition Tuberculosis (Tb)

The chest x-ray shows advanced changes of bilateral reactivation Tb, with cavitation in the upper lobes (classic location for Tb reactivation).

Pathophysiology

Tuberculosis is due to infection with *Mycobacterium tuberculosis,* an **acid-fast bacillus** spread via respiratory droplets. Tb is seen in specific populations in the U.S., including **immigrants** (especially Hispanics, Haitians, Southeast Asians), **HIV-positive patients, urban dwellers** (e.g., **New York city**), the **elderly** (who were exposed during their youth, when Tb was more prevalent) and those who **live** or **work** in **confined or high-risk areas** (e.g., prisons, nursing homes, hospitals).

Initial Tb infection is often **asymptomatic,** but Tb can **reactivate** to cause classic tuberculosis in the upper lung fields. Spread throughout the body can occur (**miliary Tb**) and nearly any organ can be involved in this setting.

Diagnosis & Treatment

Classic symptoms include a **productive cough** (often minimal), **hemoptysis** (often **blood-streaked sputum**), **night sweats,** malaise, and **weight loss**. On exam, watch for low-grade **fever** and **upper lobe rales**.

Diagnosis can be complicated. Initial measures include **respiratory isolation** and **acid-fast sputum smears,** which are specific but not sensitive. **Tuberculin (PPD) skin tests** are more sensitive, but not specific (can be positive from prior exposure without active disease or due to prior immunization, which is not done in the U.S.). In addition, some with severe disease have cutaneous **anergy** to Tb (no reaction). The definition of a positive test is ≥ **5 mm** of **palpable skin induration 48–72 hours after dermal injection of PPD** in those at **high** risk (HIV/immunosuppression, recent Tb contact, suspect Tb on chest x-ray); ≥ **10 mm** in those at **intermediate** risk (live in/come from high prevalence area, extremes of age, diabetics); and ≥ **15** mm in the **general population**. The gold standard for diagnosis is **culture,** which can take **6–8 weeks**. Polymerase chain reaction is used with a positive acid-fast smear to yield a faster diagnosis.

In PPD-positive patients *without* clinical evidence of active disease (i.e., a screening PPD done in a high-risk patient), treatment is **isoniazid** monotherapy for 6 months. **Active disease** is initially treated with **three or four** drugs, including isoniazid, **rifampin**/rifabutin, and **pyrazinamide,** with **ethambutol** or streptomycin added for suspected multidrug-resistant Tb. **Directly observed therapy** (watch the patient take pills) is usually advised.

More High-Yield Facts

Screen all high-risk persons (e.g., HIV positive, nursing home residents).

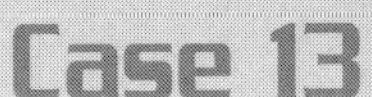

Case 13

Internal Medicine

History

A 36-year-old man is experiencing excessive daytime sleepiness that has begun to impair his work performance. He says he has fallen asleep at his desk unintentionally several times during work. The patient has tried taking scheduled naps, but these do not seem to alleviate his sleepiness. He claims he gets 8 to 10 hours of sleep per night, but often wakes up in the morning feeling more tired than he did before going to sleep. In addition, he frequently wakes up in the morning with headaches and mentions that his wife is constantly complaining about his snoring.

The patient has no significant past medical history and takes no regular medications. He drinks alcohol roughly 5 nights per week and smokes one-half pack of cigarettes per day. He is sexually active only with his wife, but says his sex drive has been rather low over the past several months. The patient denies depression or suicidal ideation.

Exam

T: 98.2°F BP: 144/90 RR: 16/min. P: 86/min.

The patient is obese but in no acute distress. Oral examination reveals a narrow posterior oropharynx. His neck is short and thick, but no adenopathy is noted. Chest and abdominal exams are normal. The rest of the exam is unremarkable.

Tests

Hemoglobin: 18 mg/dL (normal 14–18)
White blood cell count: 7000/μL (normal 4500–11,000)
Platelets: 280,000/μL (normal 150,000–400,000)
Sodium: 139 meq/L (normal 135–145)
Potassium: 4.2 meq/L (normal 3.5–5)
BUN: 10 mg/dL (normal 8–25)
Creatinine: 1 mg/dL (normal 0.6–1.5)
Glucose, fasting: 105 mg/dL (normal fasting 70–110)

Obstructive sleep apnea (OSA)

Pathophysiology

OSA is a common disorder characterized by repeated episodes of upper airway collapse and obstruction, resulting in **temporary hypoxia** and sleep disturbance. OSA has been linked to **hypertension, car accidents,** increased medical care usage, and **neuropsychiatric impairment**.

Risk factors include **increasing age** (the typical patient is a **middle-aged male**), **obesity, alcohol/sedative use, smoking,** and **anatomic upper airway narrowing** of any cause (e.g., deviated nasal septum, enlarged tongue, enlarged tonsils/adenoids).

Diagnosis & Treatment

The classic symptoms are **chronic (often loud) snoring** and **excessive daytime sleepiness**. Other common symptoms include **frequent nighttime awakening, unrefreshing sleep** (patients often report waking up more tired than they were before they went to sleep), and **headaches** upon waking. Episodes of **choking or apnea during sleep** may be reported by those who sleep with the affected person. Other possible symptoms include **memory disturbances, irritability, depression,** and **decreased libido**.

Examination of the patient with OSA classically reveals **obesity,** a **short, thick neck,** and a crowded-appearing or **narrow posterior oropharynx. Hypertension** is common and is often related to OSA. Secondary **polycythemia** may be present in severe cases (a reaction to repeated episodes of hypoxia). Severe OSA can lead to **right heart failure** (**cor pulmonale**). The diagnosis should be confirmed with **polysomnography** (sleep study), which can detect episodes of apnea and oxygen desaturations.

Treatment is initiated with **conservative measures** (e.g., **weight loss,** alcohol and smoking cessation). **Nasal continuous positive airway pressure** is the mainstay of therapy if conservative measures fail. The device creates positive pressure that "splints" open the airway, **preventing collapse**/obstruction. Oral appliances or surgery are helpful in select cases.

More High-Yield Facts

An arterial blood gas performed on an OSA patient during the day may reveal a **metabolic alkalosis**. This is because episodes of hypoxia/hypercapnia during sleep cause a respiratory acidosis. The body adjusts by retaining bicarbonate (**compensatory** metabolic alkalosis). During the day, the patient breathes well; thus the metabolic alkalosis is no longer compensating for anything and becomes the **primary** disturbance.

Case 14

Internal Medicine

History

A 66-year-old woman complains of pain in the joints of her hands. She says she has had "arthritis" for the last 5 years, though she has never seen a doctor about it and made the diagnosis herself. The patient's pain occurs in the fingers of both hands, especially after gardening and in the evenings. She finally decided to come see you because she has required increasing amounts of aspirin, which upset her stomach. The patient also wants you to look at some "bumps" on her fingers, to make sure they are not cancer. She denies fever and skin swelling or erythema over the affected joints.

Her past medical history is unremarkable and she takes no other medications. She does not smoke and only drinks on rare social occasions. The patient denies any family history of arthritis.

Exam

T: 98.2°F BP: 134/86 RR: 14/min. P: 76/min.

The patient is healthy appearing, and no skin lesions are noted. Her physical exam is entirely within normal limits, except for her hands. When asked to point to specific areas that bother her, the patient points to her distal and proximal interphalangeal joints. These joints are not erythematous; do not have increased temperature or overlying skin swelling; and are nontender to palpation. The bumps that the patient is concerned about are smooth, bony, hard nodularities located on both the medial and lateral aspects of the distal interphalangeal joints (see figure).

Tests

Hemoglobin: 14 mg/dL (normal 12–16)
White blood cell count: 6700/μL (normal 4500–11,000)
Platelets: 240,000/μL (normal 150,000–400,000)
Creatinine: 1 mg/dL (normal 0.6–1.5)
Glucose, fasting: 85 mg/dL (normal fasting 70–110)
Erythrocyte sedimentation rate: 8 mm/hr (normal 1–20)

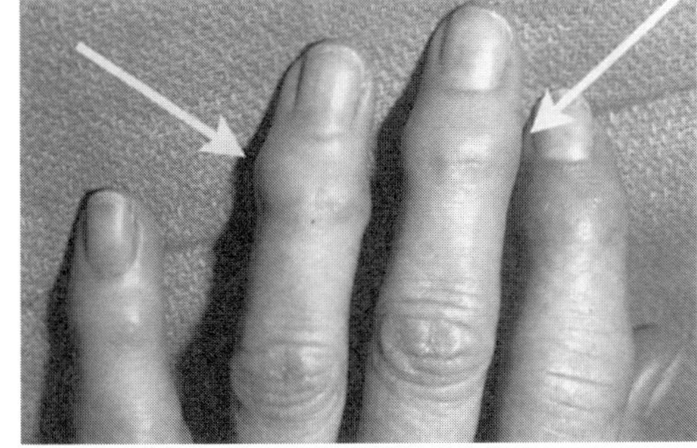

From Mangione S (ed): Physical Diagnosis Secrets. Philadelphia, Hanley & Belfus, Inc., 2000, pp 479–493; with permission.

Condition

Osteoarthritis (OA)

The photo shows **Heberden's nodes** of the **distal interphalangeal joints,** which are due to **osteophyte** (bony outgrowth or protuberance) **formation**.

Pathophysiology

OA (degenerative joint disease) is one of the **most common chronic medical disorders** known. It affects almost everyone **over age 65** to some extent, even when asymptomatic. Many cases are idiopathic and attributed to "wear and tear" of everyday living, but some cases result from **bony or metabolic abnormalities, prior trauma,** or a **neuropathic** (Charcot) joint. The most common risk factors are **increasing age** and **obesity**.

Diagnosis & Treatment

Classic symptoms of OA occur in older individuals and **progress gradually**. Commonly affected joints include the **interphalangeal joints of the hands, as well as the knees, hips,** and **spine**. Symptoms classically **worsen in the evening** and **after using the affected joints** (versus rheumatoid arthritis, which often causes morning stiffness and improved symptoms with use). The joints are characteristically **not inflamed** in OA (**no joint effusion, erythema, heat or overlying skin swelling**), separating OA from most other types of arthritis. Constitutional symptoms (fever, malaise, weight loss) are *absent*.

On exam, affected joints are **nontender**. Heberden's (more common) or **Bouchard's** (proximal interphalangeal osteophytes) **nodes** are classic in the hand. X-rays reveals **joint-space narrowing, sclerosis,** and osteophyte formation, though the severity of symptoms and the x-ray findings may not correlate. If joint fluid is aspirated (*unnecessary* in most cases), the white blood cell count will be *low,* with a *low* percentage of neutrophils and *absence* of bacteria or crystals.

Initial treatment is **acetaminophen** or **aspirin/NSAIDs**. Those with gastrointestinal problems (e.g., ulcers, bleeding) from NSAIDs can be given a **COX-II inhibitor** (e.g., celecoxib, rofecoxib) or a **diclofenac/misoprostol** preparation. Severe cases unresponsive to medical therapy may require surgery (**arthroplasty,** usually prosthetic knee or hip replacement).

More High-Yield Facts

Other drugs for OA include tramadol, capsaicin cream (thought to deplete substance P), intra-articular corticosteroid injections (no more than one injection every 3 months), and intra-articular hyaluronic acid injections.

The **pediatric hip disorders** (congenital hip dysplasia, Legg-Calvé-Perthes disease, and slipped capital femoral epiphysis) are classic causes of early-onset OA.

Case 15

Internal Medicine

History

A 33-year-old woman seeks medical advice for generalized muscle pain and aches of 3-month duration, as well as morning muscle stiffness and severe fatigue unrelieved by sleep and rest. The patient has missed work several times in the last month because her pain and fatigue made her unable to work. She has been to see another doctor that "did a bunch of blood tests, then told me it was all in my head." She is coming to you for a second opinion. The patient denies depression or depressive symptoms, but says she has become frustrated by the duration and severity of her symptoms. She has no significant past medical history and takes only as-needed acetaminophen for pain relief. She does not smoke, drink alcohol, or use illicit drugs.

Exam

T: 98.7°F BP: 124/80 RR: 14/min. P: 70/min.

The patient is thin and in no acute distress. Eye, ear, nose, and throat exam is normal, and skin lesions and lymphadenopathy are absent. Chest, abdomen, pelvic, rectal, and neurologic exams are also normal. Musculoskeletal exam reveals multiple, fairly focal, bilateral areas of increased tenderness in the posterior cervical region, upper and lower back, gluteal region, adjacent to the elbows, and behind the knees.

Tests

Hemoglobin: 14 mg/dL (normal 12–16)
White blood cell count: 6500/μL (normal 4500–11,000)
Platelets: 270,000/μL (normal 150,000–400,000)
Creatinine: 1 mg/dL (normal 0.6–1.5)
Glucose, fasting: 85 mg/dL (normal fasting 70–110)
Thyroid-stimulating hormone (TSH): 3 μU/mL (normal 0.5–5)
Erythrocyte sedimentation rate (ESR): 8 mm/hr (normal 1–20)
Antinuclear antibody titer: negative
Rheumatoid factor: negative
Creatine phosphokinase (CPK): 25 u/L (normal 17–148)

Fibromyalgia

Pathophysiology

Fibromyalgia is an idiopathic disorder characterized by chronic muscular pain in the *absence* of an identifiable organic cause. It tends to affect **middle-aged women** and is a **diagnosis of exclusion**.

Diagnosis & Treatment

Classic symptoms include **generalized muscle pain for at least 3 months, muscle stiffness** (usually in the **morning**), **fatigue,** and **sleep disturbances** (generally nonrefreshing sleep). Other symptoms that may be present include headache, subjective swelling, and depressed mood. Symptoms may **interfere with daily tasks.**

Findings include fairly **focal areas of muscular tenderness** that are often **bilateral and symmetric** in **several areas**. These areas may include the **occiput** and **back of the neck, upper and lower back, gluteal region, anterior upper ribs, elbows, and knees**. The rest of the exam and laboratory tests are *normal*. No joint effusions, reflex abnormalities, or limitation of passive range of motion should be present. At a minimum, rule out **collagen vascular disease** (with an ESR, antinuclear antibody titer, and rheumatoid factor), **hypothyroidism** (with a TSH level), **inflammatory myopathies** (with a CPK level), and **polymyalgia rheumatica** (with an ESR).

Treatment is individualized, but includes education about the condition (do *not* tell patients "It's all in your head"), support, and symptomatic treatment. No one treatment is effective for all patients. Moderate **exercise** should be encouraged. Commonly used treatments include **NSAIDs, antidepressants,** muscle relaxers, and "trigger point" muscle injections (inject local anesthetic +/− corticosteroid into muscles at point of focal tenderness). Meditation and biofeedback may also be helpful for some patients.

More High-Yield Facts

Differentiation of "polymuscle" disorders:

- Fibromyalgia—**electromyograph** (EMG), ESR, and **muscle biopsy** are all normal.
- **Polymyositis** causes an elevated ESR, **increased CPK,** and an **abnormal EMG and muscle biopsy**.
- **Polymyalgia rheumatica** causes a **markedly elevated ESR,** with a normal muscle biopsy and EMG findings. It is classically associated with temporal arteritis (though not always).

Treatment for polymyalgia rheumatica and polymyositis is **corticosteroids**.

Case 16

Internal Medicine

History

A 60-year-old man who you have followed for years is now complaining of a bad case of "the flu." His symptoms include fever, chills, night sweats, fatigue, malaise, and muscle aches. The patient says he normally wouldn't bother you, but his symptoms have persisted for 3 weeks. He also mentions a 5-pound weight loss during the course of his symptoms. He denies any sick contacts or recent travel.

Past medical history is significant only for mitral valve stenosis from childhood rheumatic fever, and arthritis. His only medication is as-needed acetaminophen. The patient does not smoke or drink alcohol. You last saw him 6 months ago for a routine check-up, which revealed no problems, and he mentions that he went to the dentist roughly a month ago for a tooth extraction and root canal procedure.

Exam

T: 101.4°F BP: 128/82 RR: 14/min. P: 104/min.

The patient appears ill and is somewhat pale. His skin is warm and flushed. Head, neck, and lung exams are remarkable only for scleral pallor. Cardiac exam reveals the patient's characteristic mitral stenosis murmur as well as a new 3/6 intensity, high-pitched, blowing, and pansystolic murmur heard best at the cardiac apex, with radiation into the axilla. Abdominal and rectal examinations are unremarkable, and the stool is negative for occult blood. You note several short, thin linear foci of hemorrhage under several fingernails. Some unusual retinal lesions are seen on funduscopic exam (see figure).

Tests

Hemoglobin: 11 mg/dL (normal 14–18)
Mean corpuscular volume (MCV): 88 μm/cell (normal 80–100)
White blood cell count: 14,100/μL (normal 4500–11,000)
Neutrophils: 82%
Platelets: 390,000/μL (normal 150,000–400,000)
Ferritin: 278 μg/L (normal 20–200)
Creatinine: 1 mg/dL (normal 0.6–1.5)
ESR: 80 mm/hr (normal 1–20)
TSH: 2.0 μU/mL (normal 0.5–5)
Antinuclear antibody titer: negative
Lipase: 9 u/dL (normal 4–24)
AST: 18 u/L (normal 7–27)

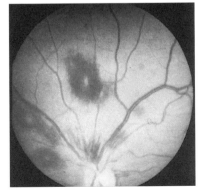

From Gold DH, Weingeist TA (eds): The Eye in Systemic Disease. Philadelphia, Lippincott, 1990, pp 3–5; with permission.

Condition Subacute bacterial endocarditis

The picture reveals **Roth spots** (white-centered retinal hemorrhages), a rare finding but one that strongly suggests bacterial endocarditis in this setting.

Pathophysiology

Most cases of endocarditis are bacterial. Bacterial endocarditis (BE) is usually classified as **acute** (classically caused by ***Staphylococcus aureus***) or **subacute** (typically caused by **viridans** or other low-virulence **streptococci**), with acute cases presenting in a more fulminant manner. Subacute cases generally involve infection of a previously **abnormal or prosthetic valve,** while acute cases involve infection of a previously **normal** valve. **Bacteremia** (from sepsis, intravenous drug abuse, or oral, bowel, or genitourinary procedures or infections) allows seeding and infection of one or more heart valves. BE is **fatal** if untreated.

Diagnosis & Treatment

The usual patient is either an **IV drug abuser** (who will typically get right-sided valvular infection, which is less common) or someone with an **abnormal or prosthetic heart valve** with a recent cause for bacteremia (a recent dental procedure is classic). Subacute BE symptoms include **fever, chills, malaise, night sweats, fatigue, arthralgias,** and **weight loss**. Septic **emboli** may cause end-organ damage/infarction symptoms (stroke, myocardial infarction, renal infarction, or lung infarction with right-sided lesions). Acute BE has similar symptoms with a **more rapid and fulminant course**. Patients may present with high fevers and **septic shock**.

Classic findings include a **new-onset heart murmur** (usually **regurgitation;** e.g., the mitral regurgitation murmur described in this case), **fever,** and **pallor** (from anemia of chronic disease in subacute cases or impending shock in acute cases). **Splinter hemorrhages** (the hemorrhages described under the fingernails), **Osler's nodes** (painful, erythematous, subcutaneous nodules in the tips of the fingers), and **Roth spots** are rare but classic findings. **Leukocytosis** with **increased neutrophils** is common, as is an **elevated erythrocyte sedimentation rate (ESR)**.

The diagnosis is confirmed with **positive blood cultures** (draw **at least three** cultures) and demonstration of **septic valvular vegetations** with **echocardiography** (transesophageal echo is more sensitive than transthoracic). Treatment is **4–6 weeks of IV antibiotics**. After cultures are drawn, broad-spectrum antibiotics are given empirically until culture results are known (e.g., ampicillin plus an aminoglycoside). **Surgery** may be needed if medical therapy fails (usually in the presence of a prosthetic valve).

More High-Yield Facts

*Fever without an obvious source plus either IV drug abuse or a new-onset heart murmur equals endocarditis **"until proven otherwise."***

Case 17

Internal Medicine

History

A 47-year-old woman is experiencing fatigue, weakness, and headaches that have gradually worsened over the past 2 months. She also mentions constipation, nausea, "feeling depressed," polyuria, and "always feeling thirsty." The patient denies suicidal ideation, weight loss, fever, and recent sick contacts. Three months ago, she felt completely healthy. Her past medical history is notable only for a "kidney stone," which she passed spontaneously 1 month ago. She takes no regular medications or vitamins and does not smoke or drink alcohol. Family history is noncontributory.

Exam

T: 98.7°F BP: 130/84 RR: 14/min. P: 84/min.

The patient is thin and in no acute distress. The sclerae are not pale, and no lymphadenopathy is appreciated. Lung and cardiac exams are unremarkable. The abdomen is not tender to palpation, but bowel sounds are hypoactive. Musculoskeletal exam reveals slight symmetric weakness in all four extremities. The remainder of the examination is normal.

Tests

Hemoglobin: 15 mg/dL (normal 12–16)
Platelets: 300,000/μL
Sodium: 142 meq/L (normal 135–145)
Calcium: 12 mg/dL (normal 8.5–10.5)
Fasting glucose: 82 mg/dL (normal 70–110)
Parathyroid hormone level:
35 pg/mL (normal < 25)
ESR: 9 mm/hr (normal 1–20)
EKG: see figure

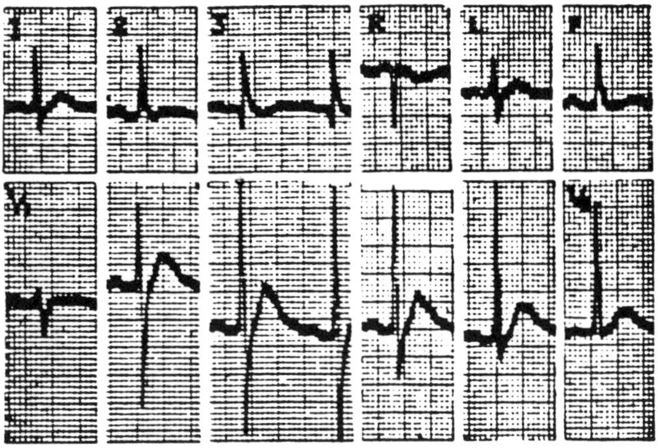

WBCs: 7400/μL
Creatinine: 1.2 mg/dL (normal 0.6–1.5)
Potassium: 3.9 meq/L (normal 3.5–5)
Albumin: 4.2 g/dL (normal 3.5–5)

From Habib GB, Zollo Jr AJ: Cardiology. Zollo Jr AJ (ed): Medical Secrets, 2nd ed. Philadelphia, Hanley & Belfus, Inc., 1997, pp 59–95; with permission.

Condition

Hyperparathyroidism

The EKG shows **QT interval shortening** with virtual absence of the ST segment.

Pathophysiology

Most cases of **hypercalcemia** are due to hyperparathyroidism (generally caused by a PTH-secreting parathyroid adenoma). **Women** are affected **three times** as often as men and the incidence increases with **age. Parathyroid hormone** (PTH) stimulates the kidney to make **1,25-vitamin D** (increasing gut absorption of calcium) and re-absorb more calcium, and also stimulates **bone resorption**. PTH also causes a **decreased** serum **phosphorus** level.

Other causes of hypercalcemia include **malignancy** (the patient usually has a known or obvious cancer in this setting, and the PTH level is *low*), **excess calcium or vitamin D intake, sarcoidosis,** and **immobilization**.

Diagnosis & Treatment

Many patients are **asymptomatic,** and the elevated calcium is discovered during routine lab work. Classic symptoms include **fatigue, lethargy, muscular aches and weakness, headaches, polyuria/polydipsia** (from impaired renal concentrating ability), **psychiatric disturbances** (e.g., **depression**), **constipation,** and **abdominal pain** (which can be nonspecific or related to renal stones, peptic ulcer disease, or pancreatitis). In fact, a classic presentation is **acute renal colic** (hypercalcemia increases renal stone risk).

Physical exam is **usually normal,** though muscular weakness may be present. The underlying cause (e.g., malignancy) may produce findings, however. EKG may reveal QT shortening. Labs generally reveal **high calcium, low phosphorus,** and **high PTH** with hyperparathyroidism (PTH is often *low* with other causes).

Initial treatment is to lower the calcium level with **hydration**. In symptomatic cases, this is generally done with IV **normal saline**. If the hypercalcemia persists, **furosemide** can be given to cause calcium diuresis. Other agents (oral phosphorus, calcitonin, diphosphonates) are sometimes needed. The definitive treatment is **surgical resection** of the adenoma. Preoperative **localization** of the adenoma can be done with a nuclear medicine scan, if desired by the surgeon.

More High-Yield Facts

Do *not* give thiazide diuretics if hypercalcemia is present (can aggravate or even cause hypercalcemia by increasing renal calcium absorption).

Mnemonic for hypercalcemia symptoms: **bones** (bone changes from resorption, now rarely seen), **stones** (kidney stones), **groans** (abdominal pain, nausea, constipation), and **psychiatric overtones** (e.g., depression, psychosis).

Case 18

Internal Medicine

History

A 27-year-old woman presents with a chief complaint of painful and frequent urination. Her symptoms began 2 days ago. The patient denies vaginal discharge or hematuria, but thinks she may have a slight fever. Past medical history is unremarkable, and the patient takes no medications. She denies any history of sexually transmitted diseases and is sexually active only with her husband of 5 years.

Exam

T: 99.8°F   BP: 120/78   RR: 14/min.   P: 74/min.

The patient is thin and healthy appearing. Her abdomen is nontender to palpation, and normal bowel sounds are present. Pelvic exam reveals no tenderness or other abnormalities. No discharge or irritation of the vagina or cervix is evident on speculum exam. The rest of the examination is normal.

Tests

Hemoglobin: 13 mg/dL (normal 12–16)
White blood cell count: 9400/μL (normal 4500–11,000)
Platelets: 310,000/μL (normal 150,000–400,000)
Creatinine: 0.9 mg/dL (normal 0.6–1.5)
Sodium: 142 meq/L (normal 135–145)
Potassium: 3.9 meq/L (normal 3.5–5)
Urinalysis: negative for glucose, protein, and bilirubin; 3+ bacteria, 2+ white blood cells (WBCs), 1+ red blood cells (RBCs), leukocyte esterase positive, nitrate positive

Condition Urinary tract infection (UTI), lower

Pathophysiology

At least 75% of non-sexually transmitted UTIs are due to ***Escherichia coli***; other gram-negative organisms and *Staphylococcus saprophyticus* are less common. **Reproductive-age females** are roughly **20–50 times** more likely to get a UTI than males the same age. This difference is thought to be due to the proximity of the short female urethra and bladder to the anus, as most bacteria are from the GI tract. Other UTI risk factors include conditions that promote **urinary stasis** (e.g., prostatic hypertrophy, neurogenic bladder, vesicoureteral reflux, pregnancy) or **bacterial colonization** (e.g., indwelling bladder catheter, fecal incontinence, surgical procedures).

Urinary tract infections are generally classified as **lower** (cystitis and urethritis; less serious) and **upper** (pyelonephritis; can be life threatening).

Diagnosis & Treatment

Classic symptoms include **dysuria,** urinary **frequency** and/or **urgency,** and **suprapubic** or **low back pain**. **Hematuria** may be present in some cases. Physical exam is normal in simple UTI, though a low-grade **fever** may be present. **High fevers, chills, nausea/vomiting, costovertebral angle tenderness,** or a **high white blood cell count** generally indicate progression to **pyelonephritis**.

Diagnosis is usually confirmed with **urinalysis,** though **urine culture** is the **gold standard** (not generally needed for simple uncomplicated cases, but mandatory for those with pyelonephritis, indwelling catheter, or other complicating factors). Urinalysis classically reveals some combination of positive **bacteria, WBCs, RBCs, nitrate,** and/or **leukocyte esterase**. The best urine sample is from catheterization of the bladder, but a **mid-stream,** "clean-catch" sample is acceptable for uncomplicated cases. **Sexually transmitted diseases,** which can cause similar symptoms, must be excluded in the appropriate setting.

Treatment is **empiric antibiotics for 3 to 5 days** with simple cystitis. **Trimethoprim-sulfamethoxazole or amoxicillin** are the best choices, though ciprofloxacin is increasingly used. Pyelonephritis is often treated on an **inpatient** basis with **IV** antibiotics after samples for urine and **blood** cultures are obtained.

More High-Yield Facts

Those in the hospital (nosocomial bugs) and with **indwelling catheters** are much more likely to have bugs other than *E. coli*.

If a young child gets UTIs, consider **congenital** urinary tract abnormalities.

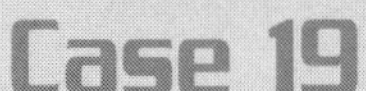

Case 19

Internal Medicine

History

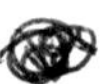

A 35-year-old woman is suffering pain and swelling in her right leg. She said her symptoms began 2 days ago, as she was getting off a plane after a 13-hour flight from overseas. Her symptoms have gradually increased since that time. She denies left leg complaints, shortness of breath, or chest pain. Past medical history is insignificant, and the patient's only regular medication is oral contraceptive pills. The patient smokes 1 pack of cigarettes per day.

Exam

T: 100.8°F BP: 132/86 RR: 12/min. P: 72/min.

The patient is obese, but in no acute distress. Her right leg below the knee is edematous, enlarged, mildly erythematous, and quite warm to the touch when compared to the left. The calf is also tender to palpation. A hard cord is palpable deep within in the popliteal fossa. With the knee flexed, forceful dorsiflexion of the knee causes severe calf pain. The rest of the physical exam is normal.

Tests

Hemoglobin: 13 mg/dL (normal 12–16)
White blood cell count: 8400/μL (normal 4500–11,000)
Platelets: 330,000/μL (normal 150,000–400,000)
Creatinine: 0.9 mg/dL (normal 0.6–1.5)
Sodium: 142 meq/L (normal 135–145)
Potassium: 3.9 meq/L (normal 3.5–5)
D-dimer: positive

Condition Deep venous thrombosis (DVT)

In this patient, the DVT is likely of the popliteal vein.

Pathophysiology

DVT is primarily of concern because it can lead to **pulmonary embolus** (PE) and **chronic venous insufficiency**. The risk factors are summarized by **Virchow's triad: endothelial damage** (e.g., trauma, infection), **stasis** of blood flow (e.g., immobilization, long airplane flight or car ride, major surgery, heart failure, obesity), and **hypercoagulable state** (e.g., oral contraceptives, genetic tendencies, malignancy, pregnancy).

Diagnosis & Treatment

Classic symptoms include **pain, swelling, increased temperature,** and **skin erythema**. Patients often have one or more risk factors for DVT. Symptoms may come on **gradually** over a few days.

Physical findings are **unreliable,** but may include the above plus calf/leg **tenderness,** a **palpable cord** in the region of a deep vein, and **Homan's sign** (dorsiflexion of the ankle with the knee flexed causes calf pain). Enlarged collateral veins may be seen in the leg in some cases. The **D-dimer** may be positive, but this is not specific and can be found in normal people. Symptoms and signs of PE may be present. The diagnosis is generally made with **imaging,** usually a Doppler venous **ultrasound**. Impedance plethysmography, standard venography, and magnetic resonance venography are other diagnostic options.

Treatment is anticoagulation with either standard or low-molecular-weight **heparin** and **warfarin**. Once warfarin causes **prothrombin time prolongation** (measured using the international normalized ratio [INR], with a goal level of roughly **2 to 3 times normal**), the heparin product can be stopped. Anticoagulation is generally advised for at least **3–6 months** after the first episode and **indefinitely** if a second episode of DVT occurs. Any **modifiable** DVT risk factors should also be addressed (e.g., stop the oral contraceptive pills). In those who are not anticoagulation candidates for any reason, a metal **filter** (e.g., Greenfield filter) can be placed inside the **inferior vena cava** to prevent PE.

More High-Yield Facts

The inherited causes of a hypercoagulable state include **factor V Leyden, thrombin variant,** and **antithrombin 3, protein C, and protein S deficiency**. These should be tested for in all patients without an obvious cause of DVT. Those who are positive often need permanent anticoagulation.

A superficial palpable cord is due to **superficial thrombophlebitis** (not DVT), which does *not* lead to PE. Treat with **aspirin** and local heat.

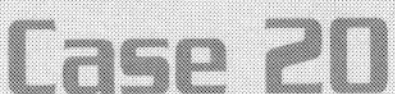

Internal Medicine

History

A 27-year-old man has been experiencing sharp, stabbing, intense chest pain for the last 24 hours. It is aggravated by deep breathing, coughing, and laying flat, and relieved by sitting up and leaning forward. The patient also reports flu-like symptoms that began as a "cold" 1 week ago. Currently, the patient says he feels as though he has a fever and has fatigue, weakness, muscle aches, and malaise. His past medical history is unremarkable, and he takes no regular medications. He drinks alcohol and smokes cigarettes "on occasion."

Exam

T: 100.9°F BP: 122/76 RR: 14/min. P: 76/min.

The patient is thin and appears to be in pain when not sitting up and leaning forward. Head, neck, and lung exams are unremarkable, though the patient refuses to inspire deeply. Cardiac exam reveals an occasional scratching sound during auscultation, but no other abnormal cardiac sounds and a normal rhythm. The rest of the examination is normal.

Tests

Hemoglobin: 15 mg/dL (normal 14–18)
Platelets: 350,000/μL
Sodium: 142 meq/L (normal 135–145)
ESR: 49 mm/hr (normal 1–20)

WBCs: 11,400/μL
Creatinine: 0.9 mg/dL (normal 0.6–1.5)
Potassium: 3.9 meq/L (normal 3.5–5)
EKG: see figure

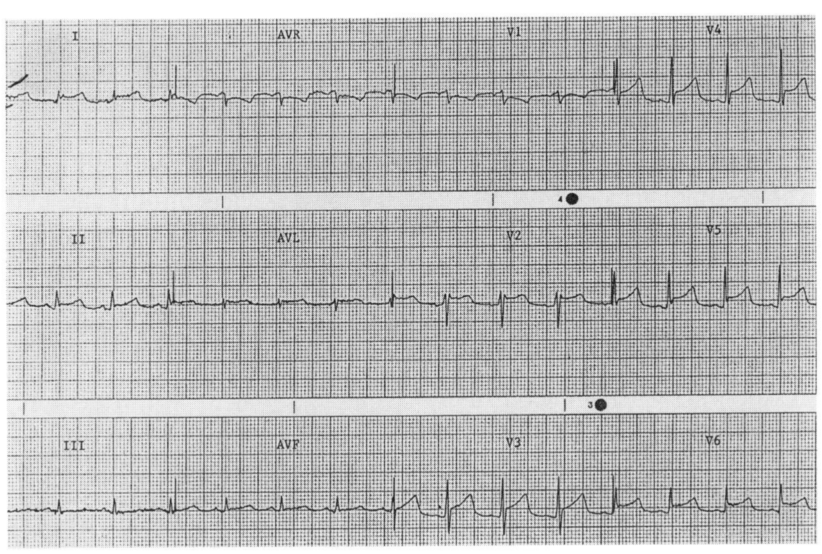

From Adair OV (ed): Cardiology Secrets, 2nd ed. Philadelphia, Hanley & Belfus, Inc., 2001, pp 139–142; with permission.

Condition Pericarditis

The EKG reveals fairly diffuse **ST segment elevation** (leads V2–V6, I, II)—a classic finding.

Pathophysiology

Most cases of pericarditis are **idiopathic** or due to **viral** causes (classically **coxsackie A or B**). Other causes can be remembered by the mnemonic **TUMOR:** trauma, uremia, myocardial infarction (e.g., Dressler's syndrome)/medications (e.g., procainamide or other lupus-causing drugs), other infections (tuberculosis, fungal, bacterial), rheumatoid arthritis and other autoimmune disorders/radiation. Inflammation of the pericardium by any of these causes can lead to pericardial effusion and/or myocarditis.

Diagnosis & Treatment

Classic symptoms include a **sharp, stabbing chest pain** that is **fairly constant** and **pleuritic** in nature (i.e., aggravated by inspiration and coughing). The pain is classically **aggravated by lying flat** and **relieved by sitting up and forward**. Other **flu-like symptoms** are common during and prior to the onset of chest pain, including cough, fever, malaise, and fatigue. Other symptoms may be produced by the underlying cause.

The classic physical finding is a **pericardial friction rub,** which is a **scratching or grating sound** heard during auscultation that usually varies with the cardiac cycle and is pathognomonic. Signs of a **pericardial effusion** may be present (e.g., muffled heart sounds, hypotension, distended neck veins), and cardiac **tamponade** can occur in some cases. Consider echocardiography in the appropriate setting. Arrhythmias or congestive heart failure can occur if **myocarditis** develops. An EKG may reveal diffuse ST elevation, and **leukocytosis, low-grade fever,** and an increased **erythrocyte sedimentation rate (ESR)** are often present. There is no one definitive confirmatory test to make the diagnosis.

Treatment is directed at the **underlying cause** (e.g., uremia, bacterial infection), when possible. In most cases, however, the cause is either viral or idiopathic, and **supportive care** and **NSAIDs/aspirin** are given to reduce symptoms until the inflammation subsides. **Corticosteroids** can be given for severe symptoms that do not subside with NSAID therapy.

More High-Yield Facts

Dressler's syndrome is pericarditis that develops roughly **1–4 weeks** after a myocardial infarction, often accompanied by fever and lasting 1–2 weeks. It is treated the same as idiopathic cases. A similar syndrome can occur after **cardiac surgery** (or any **pericardial trauma**).

Constant chest pain that lasts several hours or days is *almost never* due to ischemia. Death would likely result from ischemia of this duration.

Case 21

Internal Medicine

History

A 52-year-old man presents to the office because he is new to the area and needs a regular doctor. He has no current complaints. His past medical history is significant for hypertension and gout. The patient takes enalapril regularly and indomethacin for flares of his gout. He is unsure of his cholesterol status, but thinks it may be "a little high." The patient does not smoke and drinks alcohol on rare social occasions. Family history is noncontributory.

Exam

T: 98.8°F BP: 132/86 RR: 14/min. P: 78/min.

The patient is slightly overweight. Head, neck, chest, abdominal, and extremity exams are unremarkable. No neurologic abnormalities are detected. Given the lab information below, what recommendations would you make, if any, for managing the patient's cholesterol levels?

Tests

Total cholesterol: 232 mg/dL
LDL cholesterol: 162 mg/dL
HDL cholesterol: 28 mg/dL
Triglycerides: 210 mg/dL

Condition Elevated cholesterol for the amount of coronary artery disease (CAD) risk

Pathophysiology

To manage cholesterol levels properly, you must know a patient's CAD risk factors. There are six main risk factors: **age** (male ≥ 45, female ≥ 55), **family history** (definite myocardial infarction or sudden death in first-degree male relative < 55 or female < 65), current **cigarette smoking** (> 10 cigarettes per day or "half a pack"), **hypertension** (≥140/90 mmHg or on antihypertensive medications), **diabetes mellitus,** and a **low HDL** level (< 35 mg/dL). **HDL ≥ 60 mg/dL is protective and negates one risk factor**. Other risk factors are controversial and should *not* be used to calculate risk on the boards. High LDL and/or total cholesterol is a CAD risk factor, but is *not counted* when deciding on cholesterol treatment.

Diagnosis & Treatment

Most patients are screened with a total cholesterol level. Management details:

No CAD risk factors	≥ 2 CAD risk factors	Intervention
Total chol < 200	Total chol < 200	Remeasure in 5 years*
Total chol 200–239		Counsel and recheck in 1–2 years*
Total chol > 239	Total chol > 200	Do fasting lipoprotein analysis (gives LDL)
LDL < 160	LDL < 130	Remeasure in a year (goal met)
LDL 160–189	LDL 130–159	Diet
LDL > 189	LDL > 159	Medications

NOTE: With known CAD or peripheral vascular disease, use medications when LDL ≥ 130, with a target of LDL < 100

*Unless HDL < 35 mg/dl, in which case you should go ahead and do a full fasting lipoprotein analysis (to measure LDL)

The first intervention in all cases is **diet** (low calorie, low cholesterol), **exercise,** and **lifestyle** changes (e.g., decrease alcohol). If these measures fail after 3–6 months of trying, proceed to any other appropriate intervention. In this case, the patient has three risk factors (age, hypertension, and low HDL), so he will need medications if 3–6 months of conservative measures fail. The classic first-line agents are **bile acid sequestrants** (e.g., cholestyramine) and **niacin,** though **HMG-CoA reductase inhibitors** are now much more commonly used (better tolerated by patients).

More High-Yield Facts

Get baseline liver function tests (LFTs) and periodically monitor LFTs with HMG-CoA reductase inhibitors. Muscle pain/damage can also occur.

Case 22

Internal Medicine

History

A 62-year-old woman presents to the ED with shortness of breath and fatigue that have been gradually worsening over the past 2–3 weeks. Her breathing worsens when she lies down and improves when she sits straight up. The patient has learned to keep her back and head propped up on a pillow to allow her to fall asleep. She mentions waking up several times during the night either due to severe shortness of breath or because she has to urinate. She denies fever, sick contacts, and chest pain.

The patient's past medical history is significant for poorly controlled hypertension and a heart attack 5 years ago. She is supposed to be taking metoprolol, but admits that she ran out 2 months ago and never refilled her prescription. The patient does not smoke or drink alcohol.

Exam

T: 98.8°F BP: 152/94 RR: 22/min. P: 102/min.

The patient is overweight and dyspneic at rest. Head and neck exams are unremarkable. Lung exam reveals rales in the lower one-third of the chest bilaterally. Cardiac exam reveals tachycardia and a left-sided S3 heart sound. Abdominal, pelvic, and extremity exams are unremarkable, except for 1+ pitting edema in the lower extremities.

Tests

Hemoglobin: 15 mg/dL (normal 12–16)
Creatinine: 1.3 mg/dL (normal 0.6–1.5)
Potassium: 3.9 meq/L (normal 3.5–5)
Sodium: 134 meq/L (normal 135–145)
WBCs: 8400/μL
Blood urea nitrogen: 28 mg/dL (normal 8–25)
EKG: normal sinus rhythm with evidence of left-ventricular hypertrophy
Chest x-ray: see figure

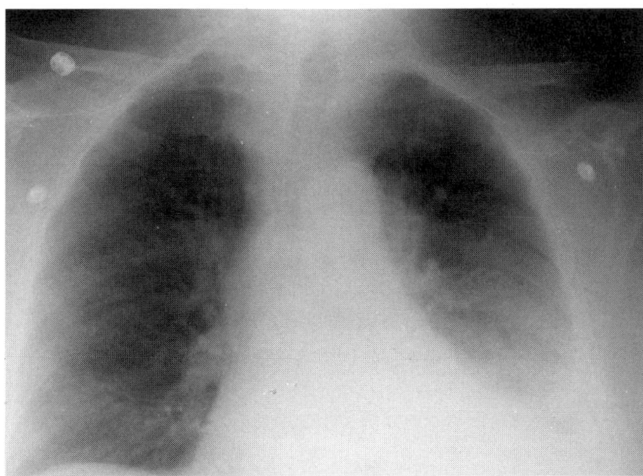

From Sahn SA, Heffner JE: Pulmonary Pearls II. Philadelphia, Hanley & Belfus, Inc., 1995, p 277; with permission.

Condition Congestive heart failure (CHF)

The chest x-ray shows cardiomegaly, pulmonary edema, and a left-sided pleural effusion.

Pathophysiology

CHF is "pump" failure and is most often due to the long-standing effects of **hypertension** and/or **coronary artery disease** (CAD). Other causes include **myocardial infarction, arrhythmias, myocarditis, anemia** (high-output failure), **hypertensive emergency, thyrotoxicosis, tamponade,** and **pulmonary embolus**. CHF can be either "left-sided" (left ventricular failure [LVF]) or "right-sided" (RVF), though **often both ventricles** are involved (the most common cause of RVF is LVF). **Cor pulmonale** is right heart enlargement/hypertrophy/failure due to lung disease (e.g., chronic obstructive pulmonary disease).

Diagnosis & Treatment

The classic symptoms of CHF are **fatigue** and **dyspnea** (from hypoxia). Other symptoms may help localize the failure to one "side." For example, LVF usually results in **orthopnea** and **paroxysmal nocturnal dyspnea,** while RVF usually causes **peripheral edema** and **nocturia**. Patients often have a cardiac history or CAD risk factors.

On exam, the classic finding of LVF is **bilateral pulmonary rales** in the lung bases. RVF may cause **jugular venous distension** and **peripheral edema**. The **S3** or **S4** heart sound is classic on cardiac auscultation and can be right- or left-sided. X-ray and EKG findings are often present, and **pre-renal azotemia** and **hyponatremia** may be found on labs. Always check **thyroid function tests** and get an EKG to rule out **myocardial infarction** or **arrhythmias**.

Initial treatment involves **oxygen** and **loop diuretics** (e.g., furosemide) for quick diuresis. In severe cases, intubation and **IV sympathomimetics** (e.g., dobutamine) may also be needed. **Sodium restriction** and an **ACE-inhibitor** should be started for the long-term, and a **beta-blocker** added once the patient is stable. Patients with more severe, stable heart failure may also need **spironolactone, furosemide,** and/or **digitalis**. Arterial and venous vasodilators (e.g., hydralazine and nitroglycerin) are other options to reduce afterload and preload, respectively. Treat other aggravating factors (e.g., hypertension, CAD risk factors) as well.

More High-Yield Facts

A previously stable CHF patient with an exacerbation of symptoms has a myocardial infarction ***"until proven otherwise,"*** even though noncompliance is the most common cause of an exacerbation.

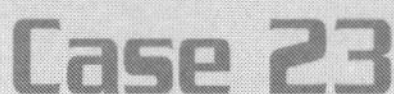

Case 23

Internal Medicine

History

A 48-year-old, homeless alcoholic is brought to the emergency department (ED) by ambulance. A friend called emergency services because the patient "seemed shaky." En route to the hospital, the emergency technicians gave the man IV normal saline and glucose. The technicians report that he has become increasingly confused since they arrived at the hospital. The patient is unable to answer questions appropriately. He is a severe alcoholic who has had withdrawal seizures in the ED on past visits.

Exam

T: 99.1°F BP: 132/84 RR: 14/min. P: 88/min.

The patient is confused and disheveled, and appears malnourished. He smells of alcohol and is lethargic, apathetic, and inattentive. Ocular exam reveals horizontal nystagmus and paralysis of lateral gaze bilaterally. Other cranial nerves are intact. Chest exam is unremarkable. The patient has mildly tender hepatomegaly, but the abdominal exam is otherwise unremarkable. On neurologic exam, the patient has a markedly ataxic gait and stance, requiring assistance to walk.

Tests

Hemoglobin: 12 mg/dL (normal 14–18)
Mean corpuscular volume: 90 μm/cell
White blood cell count: 6500/μL (normal 4500–11,000)
Platelets: 120,000/μL (normal 150,000–400,000)
Creatinine: 1.1 mg/dL (normal 0.6–1.5)
Blood urea nitrogen: 12 mg/dL (normal 8–25)
Sodium: 134 meq/L (normal 135–145)
Potassium: 4.2 meq/L (normal 3.5–5)
AST: 72 u/L (normal 7–27)
ALT: 34 u/L (normal 1–21)
Urine drug screen: negative

Condition Wernicke's encephalopathy

The patient also has alcoholic hepatitis, with the classic AST:ALT ratio of at least 2:1.

Pathophysiology

Wernicke's encephalopathy and **Korsakoff's syndrome**/psychosis are felt to be the acute and chronic sequelae, respectively, of thiamine deficiency. Both are usually seen in **malnourished alcoholics,** as most diets contain adequate thiamine. Damage to the **mamillary bodies** and thalamic nuclei may occur and are partly responsible for the clinical findings. Wernicke's is often **reversible** when treated; Korsakoff's is **irreversible**.

Diagnosis & Treatment

The classic triad of Wernicke's is **confusion** (apathy, inattention, lethargy, and slurred, irrational speech are classic), **ocular abnormalities** (**nystagmus, paralysis of lateral or conjugate gaze**), and **ataxia** (usually in the form of severe gait disturbance). Signs of alcohol withdrawal are also commonly present. Wernicke's may be confused with delirium tremens (as well as **hypoglycemia,** which can be caused by alcohol), but only patients with Wernicke's have the ocular findings. Korsakoff's syndrome is characterized by **anterograde amnesia** (can't form new memories) and **confabulation** (lying/making things up) to cover up for the amnesia.

Treatment is **IV thiamine** followed by oral supplements, and treatment of underlying withdrawal symptoms (with **benzodiazepines**) if present. Correction of **electrolyte abnormalities** is also commonly needed (hyponatremia, hypokalemia, hypomagnesemia).

More High-Yield Facts

Giving glucose to an alcoholic who has borderline thiamine deficiency can precipitate Wernicke's encephalopathy. **Give thiamine before glucose** in an alcoholic to prevent this from happening.

Alcohol abuse is associated with cancers of the **oral cavity, pharynx, esophagus,** and **liver**. It may also be associated with gastric, colon, and pancreatic cancer.

Alcohol is involved in roughly 50% of fatal **car accidents,** 67% of **drownings,** 67% of **homicides,** 35% of **suicides,** and 70–80% of deaths caused by **fire**.

Other random evils associated with alcohol: **cirrhosis, varices, gastritis, Mallory-Weiss tears, pancreatitis, anemia, thrombocytopenia, peripheral neuropathy, dilated cardiomyopathy, rhabdomyolysis, teratogenicity** (fetal alcohol syndrome), and **cerebellar degeneration**.

Case 24

Internal Medicine

History

A 27-year-old man complains of intermittent abdominal cramping, flatulence, and diarrhea of 3-week duration. The patient describes the diarrhea as watery, profuse, and foul-smelling, and says it seems to float in the toilet. He says his symptoms began shortly after returning from a week-long hiking trip in Colorado. The patient denies fever, sick contacts, tick bites, and skin rash. Prior to 3 weeks ago, he had no gastrointestinal problems. His past medical history is unremarkable, and he takes no regular medications.

Exam

T: 98.5°F BP: 122/76 RR: 12/min. P: 64/min.

The patient is thin and healthy appearing. Head, neck, chest, and extremity exams are unremarkable. Abdominal exam reveals normal bowel sounds and no tenderness to palpation. No masses are appreciated. Rectal exam reveals stool that is negative for occult blood.

Tests

Hemoglobin: 14 mg/dL (normal 14–18)
White blood cell (WBC) count: 6800/μL (normal 4500–11,000)
Platelets: 260,000/μL (normal 150,000–400,000)
Sodium: 138 meq/L (normal 135–145)
Potassium: 4 meq/L (normal 3.5–5)
AST: 12 u/L (normal 7–27)
Stool analysis: increased fat and the presence of an organism (see figure)

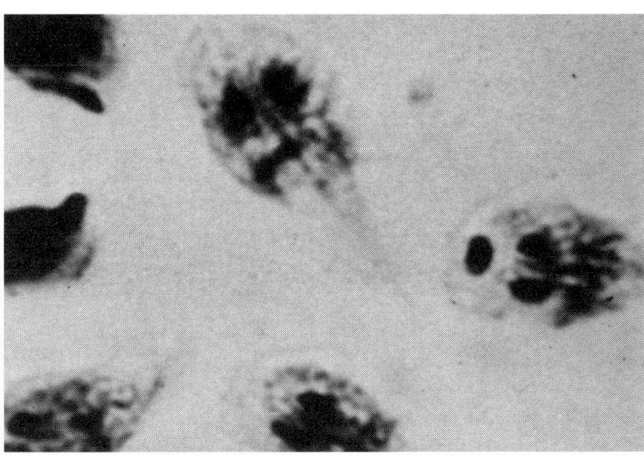

From Craft JC. In Hoeprich PD, Jordan MC (eds): Infectious Diseases, 4th ed. Philadelphia, Lippincott, 1989, pp 736–741; with permission.

Condition

Giardiasis

The figure shows the typical appearance of *Giardia lamblia* trophozoites, which are motile.

Pathophysiology

G. lamblia is a parasite transmitted via **fecally contaminated food and water** (e.g., hikers, those exposed to contaminated water sources) and the **fecal-oral route** (e.g., children in daycare centers, homosexual men). After being ingested, *G. lamblia* attaches to the wall of the **upper small bowel** and causes mucosal inflammation that can lead to **malabsorption** and other symptoms.

Diagnosis & Treatment

Classic symptoms include **non-bloody, foul-smelling, profuse, often watery or mucus-containing diarrhea** that **floats** in the toilet. These symptoms may be accompanied by **crampy abdominal pain, flatulence, nausea,** and even weight loss in severe cases. Symptoms can last for weeks or months, and fever is characteristically *absent.*

Physical findings are generally *absent*. **Stool analysis** often reveals the characteristic trophozoites and/or cysts, though several samples may need to be tested in some cases due to **intermittent shedding**. In addition, **increased fat content** of the stool (**steatorrhea**) is seen, a hallmark finding of malabsorption that is nonspecific but suggests an **upper small intestinal** process. Blood and increased WBCs are generally *not* present in the stool.

Treatment is **metronidazole** for 5–10 days. **Furazolidone** is an alternative sometimes used in children.

Preventative measures include using **filtered or purified water** when traveling or hiking, good **personal hygiene** (e.g., hand washing), and the use of **condoms** by homosexual men.

More High-Yield Facts

Giardiasis should be in the differential for any patient that presents with symptoms that remind you of **irritable bowel syndrome**. If the question on Step 2 mentions **recent onset** (as opposed to a chronic pattern of bowel complaints) or hiking, think of *Giardia.*

Endoscopy with biopsy can detect *G. lamblia* trophozoites in difficult cases. The "**string test**" is less commonly used, but involves having the patient swallow a weighted string until it reaches the duodenum, then pulling the string out. *Giardia,* if present, will adhere to the string and can be visualized.

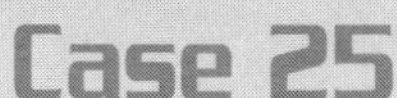

Case 25

Internal Medicine

History

A 32-year-old man would like to lose weight and he asks you if there are any medications that might help him. The patient also asks what a body mass index is and what his should be, as he saw a program on it last night. He says he has been overweight since childhood. His past medical history is unremarkable, though he was told a few years ago that he had "borderline diabetes." He currently takes no medications and does not smoke, drink alcohol, or use illicit drugs. Family history is significant for obesity and heart disease.

Exam

T: 98.7°F BP: 132/86 RR: 16/min. P: 84/min.

The patient is obese. He weighs 330 pounds (150 kg) and is 5 feet 6 inches (1.7 meters) tall. Head, neck, chest, and abdominal exams are unremarkable. No skin lesions are appreciated. Neurologic and extremity exams are normal.

Tests

Hemoglobin: 16 mg/dL (normal 14–18)
White blood cell count: 6100/μL (normal 4500–11,000)
Platelets: 280,000/μL (normal 150,000–400,000)
Sodium: 139 meq/L (normal 135–145)
Potassium: 4.1 meq/L (normal 3.5–5)
AST: 22 u/L (normal 7–27)
Glucose, fasting: 118 mg/dL (normal fasting 70–110)

Condition

Morbid obesity

The patient's **body mass index (BMI)** is roughly 52 (see below for BMI formula).

Pathophysiology

Obesity is a chronic **multifactorial** disorder with a definite **genetic component** that is now estimated to affect **one-third** of the U.S. adult and adolescent population. Obesity causes **multiple health consequences,** including an increased risk of all of the following conditions: **mortality, insulin resistance and diabetes, hypertension, hypertriglyceridemia, heart disease** and **coronary artery disease, gallstones, sleep apnea, osteoarthritis, thromboembolism, varicose veins,** and **cancer** (especially **endometrial** cancer in women).

Diagnosis & Treatment

Morbid obesity is not difficult to recognize, but you should know the definition of obesity for the boards. The BMI is currently favored to define obesity. The formula is:

$$(\text{weight in kilograms})/(\text{height in meters})^2$$

A BMI **> 25** kg/m^2 is considered "overweight," while a BMI **> 27.5** kg/m^2 defines obesity. A BMI **≥ 40** kg/m^2 is considered morbid obesity. The higher the BMI, the greater the health risks.

Initial assessment with a complete blood count, chemistry panel, and thyroid function tests should help rule out the **rare** (< 5%) cases of **organic obesity,** such as those due to **Cushing's syndrome** or **hypothyroidism**. **Screen for depression,** because it is more prevalent in obese individuals and also makes treatment more difficult.

Treatment is **gradual** weight loss through **diet and behavior modifications** as well as **regular exercise**. Drastic or starvation diets can be **dangerous** and lead to a **high relapse rate**. **Be conservative on the boards,** especially initially. In those who are morbidly obese, pharmacotherapy (e.g., orlistat) and bariatric surgery (e.g., vertical gastric banding) are sometimes considered in selected patients if initial measures fail to show any progress after several months. Exercise should begin **gradually,** with a goal of at least **30 minutes of aerobic activity 4–5 times per week**.

More High-Yield Facts

Even a **modest (10%) weight loss** can have **significant benefit,** and implementing long-term, healthy lifestyle changes is *more important* than the specific amount of weight loss within a certain time frame. If a patient loses less than you had hoped after 6 months, but is eating better and exercising regularly, do *not* change your management right away, as this is definite progress (better than most).

Case 26

Internal Medicine

History

A 37-year-old woman comes into your office complaining of worsening fatigue and blurry vision over the past few weeks. She also mentions vaginal burning and that she has been quite thirsty lately, but whatever she drinks seems "to go right through" her. The patient denies fever, sick contacts, cough, headache, diarrhea, and depression. Her past medical history is noncontributory, and she takes no regular medications. She does not smoke or drink alcohol. Family history is notable for diabetes, hypertension, and heart disease.

Exam

T: 99°F BP: 112/70 RR: 18/min. P: 108/min.

The patient is obese and mildly dyspneic. Her visual acuity is 20/60 bilaterally, and funduscopic exam reveals no abnormalities. The patient's mucous membranes are quite dry, and skin tenting is present. The chest is clear to auscultation; no cardiac murmurs are heard. Her abdomen is nontender. Pelvic exam reveals no masses. Speculum exam shows a thick, white discharge; after a potassium hydroxide preparation, hyphae are visible under the microscope. When you ask the patient to stand up at the end of the exam, she complains of feeling light-headed.

Tests

Hemoglobin: 16 mg/dL (normal 12–16)
White blood cell count: 8100/μL (normal 4500–11,000)
Platelets: 320,000/μL (normal 150,000–400,000)
Sodium: 130 meq/L (normal 135–145)
Potassium: 4.1 meq/L (normal 3.5–5)
Creatinine: 1.2 mg/dL (normal 0.6–1.5)
BUN: 28 mg/dL (normal 8–25)
Serum ketones: negative
AST: 22 u/L (normal 7–27)
Glucose: 618 mg/dL (normal fasting 70–110)
Urinalysis: positive for glucose; negative for ketones, bilirubin, protein, and bacteria

Condition Diabetes mellitus (DM), type II, new onset

Pathophysiology

DM type II accounts for **90%** of cases of DM and is generally due to **insulin resistance**. The amount of endogenous insulin secretion may be low, normal, or high compared to normal persons, but those affected have a deficiency of insulin relative to their needs. DM type II is closely associated with **obesity,** which is present in at least 75% of patients.

Diabetes causes immediate and long-term health risks. In the short term, hyperglycemia can lead to a **hyperosmolar hyperglycemic state,** which can lead to marked dehydration and even **death**. Long term, DM is a common cause of **end-stage renal disease, blindness, atherosclerosis, sensory** and **autonomic neuropathy,** and an **increased risk of infections**.

Diagnosis & Treatment

The classic presenting symptoms of new-onset or poorly controlled DM type II occur in an obese person and include **fatigue, polyuria, polydipsia, and polyphagia**. **Blurry vision** is also classic, as hyperglycemia can lead to lens swelling that can cause **myopia**. A **yeast infection** (e.g., vaginitis, thrush) may be present. **Family history** is often positive for DM.

Physical findings include **dehydration** (dry mucous membranes, skin tenting, delayed capillary refill, tachycardia, orthostatic hypotension, BUN:creatinine ratio > 15:1), and possibly **myopia** or a **yeast infection**. Labs reveal **hyperglycemia, glucosuria,** "false" **hyponatremia** (secondary to the hyperglycemia, treatment of the blood glucose normalizes the sodium level), and *absent* ketone formation (seen in type I DM with ketoacidosis).

Initial treatment includes large amounts of **intravenous fluids** (normal saline) to correct dehydration, monitoring and replacement of other **electrolytes,** and **intravenous insulin**. Once the blood sugar is brought under control, long-term management should be started. **Education and counseling** are important. **Oral medications** are the mainstay of initial therapy in most cases of type II DM. Initial regimens may include a **sulfonylurea** (including repaglinide, a sulfonylurea-like drug), **metformin, insulin sensitizers** (e.g., pioglitazone, rosiglitazone), and agents that **inhibit glucose absorption** (e.g., acarbose, miglitol). Multiple agents may be needed, and some patients will also require insulin.

More High-Yield Facts

Screen at-risk individuals with a fasting glucose level. If ≥ **126** mg/dL (or a random glucose is **> 200** mg/dL), DM is present. If the level is 110–125 mg/dL, the person is considered to have **impaired** glucose tolerance. Consider **formal testing** with an oral glucose load test, and closely monitor.

Case 27

Internal Medicine

History

A 54-year-old man is experiencing severe right knee pain and swelling that began last night when he laid down to go to sleep. The pain and swelling have progressively worsened. The patient denies trauma or overuse of the knee and says he was relaxing on the couch most of the day yesterday "just watching television, eating well, and having a few beers." He denies any prior history of arthritis, fevers, or sexually transmitted diseases. Past medical history is notable only for "borderline high blood pressure," which the patient hasn't had checked in several years. He takes no regular medications, but took acetaminophen this morning, which did not effectively relieve his pain. He smokes cigarettes and drinks alcohol on a daily basis, and admits that his diet is strictly "meat and potatoes."

Exam

T: 99.5°F BP: 142/88 RR: 14/min. P: 78/min.

The patient is slightly overweight and appears uncomfortable secondary to pain. Head, neck, chest, and abdominal exams are unremarkable. The patient's right knee is swollen, tender, warm, and has a limited range of motion secondary to pain. The skin overlying the knee is erythematous. Aspiration of the knee joint is performed, and a sample of the joint fluid is viewed using polarized light microscopy (see figure).

Tests

Hemoglobin: 16 mg/dL (normal 14–18)
WBCs: 10,800/μL (normal 4500–11,000)
Platelets: 350,000/μL (normal 150,000–400,000)
Sodium: 139 meq/L (normal 135–145)
Glucose: 108 mg/dL (normal fasting 70–110)
Potassium: 4.2 meq/L (normal 3.5–5)
Uric acid: 9.2 mg/dL (normal 3–7)
Joint fluid analysis:
  WBCs 2500/μL (normal < 200);
  Neutrophils 60% (normal < 25%);
  Gram stain negative

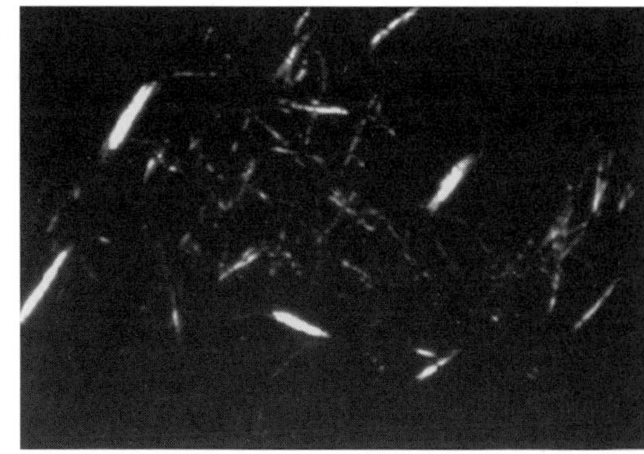

From West SG (ed): Rheumatology Secrets. Philadelphia, Hanley & Belfus, Inc., 1997, pp 265–272 ; with permission.

Condition

Gout, acute attack

Pathophysiology

Gout is a form of inflammatory arthritis due to deposition of **uric acid crystals into the joints**. It is generally associated with hyperuricemia, though this is *not* a specific finding because many people with elevated uric acid levels are asymptomatic. Risk factors include increasing **age, obesity, male sex** (male:female ratio is 3:1), **alcohol abuse,** and a **protein-rich diet**.

In most cases, gout and hyperuricemia are **primary** disorders due to **renal underexcretion** of uric acid (80–90% of primary cases) or overproduction of uric acid. **Secondary** cases can be due to purine enzyme defects, malignancy (from increased cellular and thus purine turnover), renal failure, and drugs (**aspirin** and **thiazide** diuretics are classic offenders, as they decrease renal uric acid excretion).

Diagnosis & Treatment

Acute gout classically causes a very **painful, swollen, hot, erythematous** joint. The pain typically begins at night. The most common location is the **metatarsophalangeal joint** (known as **podagra**), followed by the other foot, ankle, knee, elbow, and wrist joints. Low-grade fever and **malaise** may also be present. Hyperuricemia can also lead to **renal calculi**.

Exam reveals the above findings plus **tenderness** of the joint and a **limited range of motion** secondary to pain. In general, when an obviously inflamed joint is present (tender, swollen, hot, erythematous), **arthrocentesis** should be performed unless the diagnosis is known. Joint fluid in gout classically reveals *absence* of bacteria, **> 2000 WBC/μL** with **> 50% neutrophils,** and **uric acid crystals,** which are **needle shaped** and demonstrate **negative birefringence** with polarized light microscopy. The serum uric acid level is usually *elevated,* and **fever** and **leukocytosis** may also be present.

Initial treatment is **anti-inflammatory medications,** usually **colchicine** or **indomethacin** (not aspirin). Some patients may require additional pain medication. Once the acute attack has subsided, the goal of therapy is to **lower the uric acid level** to prevent permanent joint damage and destruction. **Allopurinol** is commonly used for this purpose, but **should be avoided during an acute attack, as it may worsen symptoms**. In addition, **weight loss, avoidance** of alcohol, and protein-rich meals are important.

More High-Yield Facts

Tophi are uric acid crystal deposits large enough to be seen on the **skin** (a **chalky, toothpaste-like material** oozing from the skin, classically seen in the hands, feet, or ears) or using **x-rays** (bones with "**punched-out**" **cystic destructive lesions** in them).

Case 28

Internal Medicine

History

A 44-year-old man is brought to the ED by his wife for confusion. The man had been complaining of headaches for the last few days, but became confused this morning, not knowing where he was and "acting funny." The patient is unable to answer questions appropriately, but his wife denies any complaints of fever, sick contacts, recent drug or alcohol use, or head trauma. She states that her husband has been well until the last few days. Past medical history is unremarkable, and he takes no regular medications. He has not seen a doctor in over 10 years. Family history is significant for hypertension in multiple first-degree relatives.

Exam

T: 98.5°F   BP: 212/120   RR: 16/min.   P: 80/min.

The patient is confused but does not appear to be in any acute distress, though he is mildly dyspneic. Funduscopic exam reveals bilateral papilledema and arteriovenous nicking, but no scleral pallor or photophobia is present. His neck is supple. Chest, abdominal, and extremity exams are unremarkable. The neurologic exam reveals difficulty concentrating, inattention, apathy, and irrational thinking, but no focal deficits.

Tests

Hemoglobin: 15 mg/dL (normal 14–18)   WBCs: 7800/μL
Sodium: 139 meq/L (normal 135–145)   Potassium: 4.9 meq/L (normal 3.5–5)
Creatinine: 1.9 mg/dL (normal 0.6–1.5)   BUN: 26 mg/dL (normal 8–25)
Urinalysis: positive for protein and microscopic hematuria;
negative for glucose, bilirubin, and bacteria
Head CT scan: normal   EKG: see figure

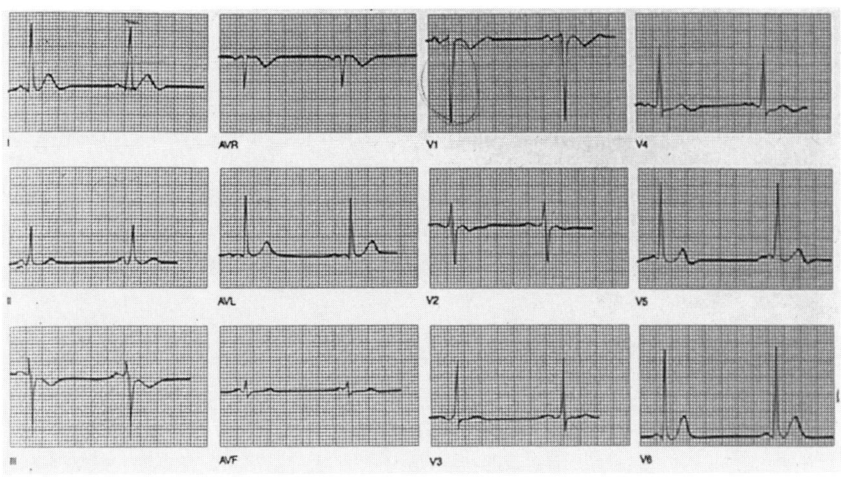

From Thaler MS. In The Only EKG Book You'll Ever Need, 3rd ed. Philadelphia, Lippincott, Williams & Wilkins, 1999, pp 61–93; with permission.

Condition Hypertensive emergency

The EKG reveals tall R waves in aVL (> 11 mm), tall R waves in V5 and V6, and deep S waves in V1 (R in V5 or V6 plus S in V1 > 35 mm), the classic findings of **left ventricular hypertrophy**.

Pathophysiology

A hypertensive emergency is defined by markedly elevated blood pressure (usually **> 210/120 mmHg**) with **acute end-organ effects** (neurologic, cardiovascular, or renal). The cause is usually idiopathic/essential hypertension, but consider **secondary** causes (e.g., pheochromocytoma).

Diagnosis & Treatment

Patients usually complain of **neurologic symptoms** (e.g., altered mental status, confusion, headaches with nausea and vomiting, dizziness, seizures, or blurry vision), or **cardiovascular symptoms** (e.g., chest pain or shortness of breath, which may be due to cardiac or renal failure). They may or may not have a personal or family **history** of hypertension.

Physical findings include **neurologic signs** (e.g., altered mental status, papilledema, positive Babinski sign, hyperreflexia) and **cardiovascular signs** (e.g., congestive heart failure or myocardial infarction). The **blood pressure is markedly elevated**. EKG and funduscopic exam (e.g., vessel "nicking" or papilledema) may reveal chronic hypertension changes (as in this case) or the EKG may show findings that suggest **acute ischemia or injury**. CT scan of the head may reveal cerebral edema, but is usually *negative*. Lumbar puncture, if performed, is *negative*. Chest x-ray may show **cardiomegaly** or **congestive failure**. Labs may demonstrate **elevated creatinine, BUN,** and **proteinuria, microscopic hematuria,** or **casts** in the urine from **necrotizing arteriolitis** in the renal vessels.

Immediate treatment is needed to prevent permanent organ damage and death. The blood pressure should be lowered in the **intensive care unit** with **short-acting intravenous** antihypertensive agents. **Nitroprusside, nitroglycerine,** or **labetalol** are commonly used. The goal is to lower the blood pressure *gradually,* trying for only a **15–25% reduction** in blood pressure over the first few hours to prevent further organ damage. Rapid lowering of the blood pressure, especially to normotensive levels, is *dangerous* and can result in acute organ **ischemia** (e.g., stroke). After initial reduction, the blood pressure can be *slowly* lowered further over the course of several days as the patient is gradually switched over to **oral medications.** Test for secondary causes of hypertension.

More High-Yield Facts

Hypertensive **urgency** is markedly elevated blood pressure *without* evidence of end-organ damage. It is treated similarly to a hypertensive emergency. In cases of markedly elevated blood pressure (> 210/120), *don't* wait for three separate blood pressure measurements to start treatment.

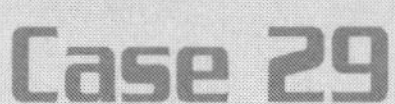

Case 29

Internal Medicine

History

A 32-year-old man comes to the office requesting a fertility evaluation. He and his wife have been trying to conceive a child for the past 4 years, unsuccessfully. They have been to see a fertility specialist, and the patient's wife has undergone extensive testing, which has revealed no abnormalities. Initially, the man refused to undergo testing due to embarrassment, but his wife has finally persuaded him to seek an evaluation. The patient admits to frequent difficulty with achieving and maintaining an erection. He has no significant past medical history, other than mild dyslexia, and takes no regular medications. The patient does not smoke, drink alcohol, or use illicit drugs. There is no family history of fertility problems.

Exam

T: 98.6°F BP: 122/78 RR: 12/min. P: 64/min.

The patient is tall and thin, with long legs and a youthful appearance; he has minimal facial and axillary hair. Bilateral, symmetric gynecomastia is found on chest exam. Genitalia exam reveals unusually small and firm testicles. No other abnormalities are identified.

Tests

Hemoglobin: 14 mg/dL (normal 14–18)
White blood cell count: 6800/μL (normal 4500–11,000)
Testosterone level: 140 ng/mL (normal 300–1100)
Follicular stimulating hormone: 28 mu/mL (normal 3–18)
Buccal smear: occasional Barr bodies

Klinefelter's syndrome

Pathophysiology

Klinefelter's syndrome generally describes individuals with a **47, XXY karyotype,** though some may have a **mosaic-type pattern** or more than two X chromosomes. The cause is most commonly **paternal meiotic nondisjunction,** or uneven chromosome distribution between dividing gametes. Patients are **psychologically and physically male,** but multiple mild **abnormalities may result** from this chromosomal disorder.

Diagnosis & Treatment

The classic presentation is for **delayed sexual development,** decreased sexual function, or **infertility,** though patients may present for unrelated complaints. On physical exam, patients are generally **tall with long legs** and have **decreased body hair** (especially **facial** and **axillary** hair). The **testes are small (< 2 cm) and firm,** and the penis may be small as well. **Gynecomastia** is another common finding. Patients may have a history of, or may demonstrate, **mild mental deficiency,** dyslexia, or social maladjustment, but frank mental retardation is *uncommon.*

Lab testing generally reveals **Barr bodies** (usually only present in women and due to the second X chromosome), **absence of sperm** in a semen sample (i.e., **azoospermia**), **decreased testosterone levels,** and **elevated gonadotropin** (i.e., follicle-stimulating hormone and luteinizing hormone) **levels**.

There is *no* satisfactory treatment, though patients that are "underandrogenized" may benefit from **testosterone** treatment. Infertility *cannot* be reversed, as the **seminiferous tubules degenerate** and/or fail to develop appropriately and are *unable* to manufacture sperm.

More High-Yield Facts

Patients with Klinefelter's syndrome have a markedly **increased risk of breast cancer** compared to normal men (though the risk is still less than it is in women).

An **XX male syndrome** also exists, and those affected are clinically similar to those with Klinefelter's syndrome, but have a **short stature** and normal intelligence.

Case 30

Internal Medicine

History

A 34-year-old woman complains of worsening fatigue, weight gain, and always feeling cold. She also mentions constipation and says that her periods have become fairly heavy recently. All of her symptoms began roughly 3 months ago and have been getting worse. She denies depression, but says, "I just don't feel like myself lately." Prior to these symptoms, the patient was healthy. She has no significant past medical history and takes no regular medications other than daily vitamins. She does not smoke, drink alcohol, or use illicit drugs.

Exam

T: 97.6°F BP: 122/88 RR: 12/min. P: 44/min.

The patient is in no acute distress. Her speech is somewhat slow, and her facial expression somewhat dull. You notice some mild periorbital puffiness of the skin, but the head and neck exams are otherwise unremarkable. Chest and abdominal exams are normal, except for bradycardia noted during the cardiac exam. Neurologic exam reveals brisk contraction during reflex testing, with a prolonged relaxation time. Tapping on the volar surface of the wrist produces tingling in several of the patient's fingertips, which she says happens spontaneously from time to time.

Tests

Hemoglobin: 10 mg/dL (normal 12–16)
Mean corpuscular volume: 88 μL/cell (normal 80–100)
White blood cell count: 7400/μL (normal 4500–11,000)
Ferritin: 130 μg/L (normal 20–200)
Total iron binding capacity: 230 μg/dL (normal 250–410)
AST: 11 u/L (normal 7–27)
Thyroid-stimulating hormone (TSH): 11 μU/mL (normal 0.5–5)
Urinalysis: negative for glucose, protein, white blood cells, and bacteria
EKG: see figure

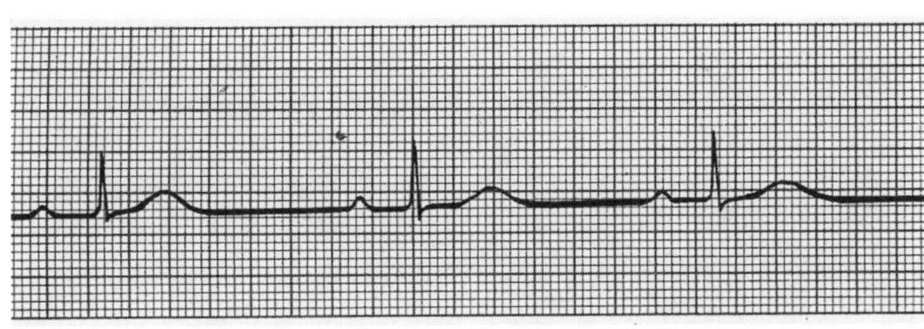

From Thaler MS. In The Only EKG Book You'll Ever Need, 3rd ed. Philadelphia, Lippincott, Williams & Wilkins, 1999, pp 95–151; with permission.

Condition Hypothyroidism

The EKG reveals sinus bradycardia (rate = 40–45/minute).

Pathophysiology

Most cases of hypothyroidism are related to **intrinsic thyroid gland dysfunction** (i.e., **primary** endocrine disturbance). Thyroid hormone has widespread effects on general metabolism and affects just about every organ system. Hypothyroidism is most commonly seen in **women of reproductive age**.

The most common cause of hypothyroidism in the U.S. is **Hashimoto's syndrome,** an autoimmune disorder that results in chronic **thyroiditis** from lymphocyte infiltration of the gland. The second most common cause is probably **treatment for hyperthyroidism** (usually Graves' disease) with radioactive thyroid ablation or surgical resection, which can destroy too much of the gland and result in hypothyroidism. Other less common causes include **drugs** (e.g., amiodarone), **postpartum thyroiditis, secondary causes** (i.e., pituitary or hypothalamic dysfunction), and the recovery phase of subacute (de Quervain's) thyroiditis.

Diagnosis & Treatment

There are many classic symptoms of hypothyroidism, including **lethargy; fatigue; cold intolerance; weight gain; depression; personality changes; coarse, dry skin; constipation;** and **menstrual disturbances** (classically menorrhagia, but amenorrhea may also occur). **Paresthesias** of the hands and feet (due to carpal or tarsal tunnel syndrome) and **facial puffiness** (especially in the periorbital region) are also classic symptoms.

The following may also be present on physical exam: **bradycardia, skin thickening,** hoarseness, slow speech, psychosis, hypothermia, **brisk contraction with delayed relaxation during reflex testing,** signs of **anemia** (often the normochromic, normocytic anemia of chronic disease), signs of **carpal tunnel syndrome,** and intellectual impairment. A **goiter** may or may not be present depending on the cause of hypothyroidism (Hashimoto's usually causes a **painless, smooth goiter**). The **TSH** is usually *elevated,* and the **triiodothyronine (T3)** and **thyroxine (T4)** levels are *decreased*. In secondary cases, the TSH is *low*.

The treatment is **thyroid replacement hormone,** often needed indefinitely, and generally given as T4. or Armour thyroid (1 grain = 9 mcg T3/38 mcg (1 grain = 100 mcg levothyroxine = 25 mcg liothyronine = 4:1 mix 1 grain).

More High-Yield Facts

In cases of Hashimoto's syndrome, **antithyroid (antimicrosomal) antibodies** are usually detectable in the serum. Other autoimmune disorders are often associated with Hashimoto's.

Levothyroxine 1.6 mcg/kg/d po qd
adjust in 12.5 to 25 mcg increments
Recheck TSH in 4-6 wk.

Case 31

Internal Medicine

History

A 20-year-old woman is experiencing sore throat, fever, malaise, and severe fatigue. She initially began noticing fatigue and malaise about 5 days ago; the fever and sore throat began yesterday. Previously the patient felt healthy. She has no significant past medical history, takes no medications, and denies any recent sick contacts. She is a student at a local college and says she drinks alcohol and smokes cigarettes "on the weekends." She is sexually active, has had two different partners in the past year, and claims to always use condoms.

Exam

T: 101.9°F BP: 118/76 RR: 14/min. P: 86/min.

The patient is athletic appearing, though she looks acutely ill. The sclera are anicteric. Throat exam reveals severe pharyngeal tenderness and erythema with a whitish-yellowish exudate. Anterior and posterior cervical adenopathy are noted on neck exam. Chest exam is unremarkable, and no cardiac murmurs are appreciated. Abdominal exam reveals a palpable spleen tip just below the left costal margin. The liver edge is also just palpable below the costal margin and is slightly tender to palpation. Normal bowel sounds are present, and no other areas of tenderness are noted. Pelvic exam, including a speculum exam, is normal. No neurologic abnormalities are present.

Tests

Hemoglobin: 12 mg/dL (normal 12–16)
White blood cell count: 12,400/µL (normal 4500–11,000)
Lymphocytes: 64%
Platelet count: 110,000/µL (normal 150,000–400,000)
Peripheral smear: multiple, heterogeneous atypical lymphocytes (see figure)
AST: 45 u/L (normal 7–27)
ALT: 48 u/L (normal 1–21)
Bilirubin, total: 1 mg/dL (normal 0.1–1.0)

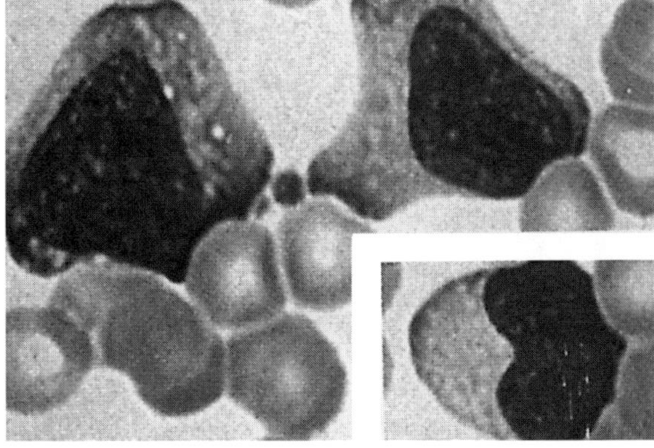

From Lee GR, et al (eds): Wintrobe's Clinical Hematology, 10th ed. Philadelphia, Williams & Wilkins, 1999, pp 1926–1955; with permission.

Condition

Infectious mononucleosis ("mono")

The photo shows the classic atypical lymphocytes.

Pathophysiology

Most cases of infectious mononucleosis (IM) are due to infection with the **Epstein-Barr virus (EBV)**. EBV is an extremely common infection: it is thought that at least half of the people in the U.S. are infected before the age of 5, when the infection is usually **asymptomatic** or causes only minimal symptoms. In those who first become infected in **late adolescence** and **early adulthood,** the classic clinical symptoms of IM often occur.

EBV has been linked to **African Burkitt's lymphoma, nasopharyngeal carcinoma,** and some **B cell lymphomas** in those who are immunocompromised. Transmission is primarily via **saliva** (IM has been called the "kissing" disease), though **blood** transmission is possible.

Diagnosis & Treatment

The classic IM tetrad is **fever, fatigue, pharyngitis,** and **lymphadenopathy**. Patients often have severe **malaise** and fatigue, followed by **sore throat** and fever. **Headaches, arthralgias,** and **anorexia** may also be present.

Physical findings include pharyngitis (which can be **exudative** and resemble streptococcal pharyngitis), adenopathy (classically symmetric cervical adenopathy), and fever. **Hepatosplenomegaly,** usually mild, may be present, and the liver may be somewhat **tender**. **Jaundice** can occur with more severe liver involvement. A maculopapular rash can be seen in some cases. Labs may reveal **leukocytosis** with a large percentage of **lymphocytes, anemia,** and/or **thrombocytopenia**. **Atypical, reactive lymphocytes** are classically present on peripheral smear and may occasionally be confused with a hematologic malignancy (but the cells are generally **heterogeneous,** making malignancy unlikely). Mild **liver enzyme elevations** are also fairly common. The diagnosis can generally be confirmed with the **IgM heterophil antibody test** (monospot test), which is positive in roughly 90% of adult cases. Specific anti-EBV antibodies (e.g., viral capsid antigen antibodies) are available in suspected cases when the monospot test is negative.

Treatment is **supportive** and symptoms generally resolve in **2–4 weeks**. Contact sports should be *avoided* temporarily to prevent splenic rupture.

More High-Yield Facts

Ampicillin + IM = maculopapular rash (develops in most people, and is not a penicillin allergy).

Consider **HIV infection** as a cause of an IM-type illness. Test if indicated.

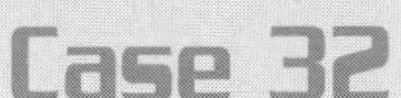

Case 32

Internal Medicine

History

A 76-year-old man complains of painful gums that bleed fairly often. He says his gums have gradually gotten worse over the past several months, but he doesn't like doctors, so he didn't see anyone about the problem. He also complains of a lack of energy, frequent pain in his shins with no history of trauma, and easy bruising. There is no history of medical problems, and he does not take medications. The patient reports that he hasn't seen a doctor in 15 years. When asked about his diet, he states: "I like my tea and toast, and that's about it."

Exam

T: 98.6°F BP: 134/86 RR: 14/min. P: 80/min.

The patient is thin and in no distress. No scleral abnormalities or adenopathy is appreciated. His gums are swollen, tender, spongy, and friable. Multiple perifollicular hemorrhages are noted in the skin in addition to follicular hyperkeratosis (see figure). There are also multiple bruises on the extremities in various stages of healing. You note dehiscence of what the patient says is an old scar on the right shoulder. Chest, abdominal, and rectal exams are normal. When a blood pressure cuff is inflated to 100 mmHg and left at this pressure for 15 minutes, an unusually large number of petechiae develop on his forearm.

Tests

Hemoglobin: 14 mg/dL (normal 14–18)
White blood cell count: 6400/μL (normal 4500–11,000)
Platelet count: 220,000/μL (normal 150,000–400,000)
Peripheral smear: normal
Creatinine: 1 mg/dL (normal 0.6–1.5)
Bleeding time: 4 minutes (normal 3–9.5 minutes)
Prothrombin time (PT): 12 seconds (normal 10–15)
Partial thromboplastin time (PTT): 28 seconds (normal 25–38)

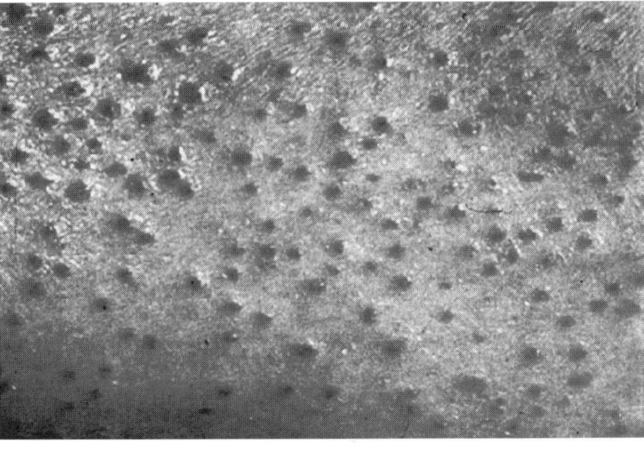

From Demidovich CW. In Fitzpatrick JE, Aeling JL (eds): Dermatology Secrets. Philadelphia, Hanley & Belfus, Inc., 1996, pp 265–268; with permission.

Condition Vitamin C deficiency (scurvy)

The photo shows **perifollicular hemorrhage** and **follicular hyperkeratosis** (nearly pathognomonic).

Pathophysiology

Vitamin C deficiency is rare in the U.S., but can be seen in the **urban poor** and the **elderly,** especially in those on **unusual diets** (classic are the "**tea and toast**" or "**hot dogs and soda**" diets in the elderly) that do *not* include fresh **fruit or vegetables**. Vitamin C is involved in **iron absorption, collagen formation** and **wound healing,** other metabolic processes, and immune function.

Diagnosis & Treatment

Look for a boards question on vitamin C deficiency to specifically mention an unusual diet or cause for severe **malabsorption**. Patients may complain of **malaise, fatigue, myalgias, arthralgias, bone pain** (due to **subperiostial bone hemorrhages**), **painful and bleeding gums, poor wound healing,** and **easy bruising**.

Physical findings include swollen, tender, **friable gums** (may be spongy and purplish in color); the skin findings shown in the photo; and **splinter hemorrhages** under the distal fingernails. Multiple bruises and **dehiscence of old scars** (or poor healing of newer wounds) may also be seen. The **capillary fragility test** is almost always abnormal. In this test, a blood pressure cuff is left inflated to a pressure midway between the systolic and diastolic pressure for 15 minutes, and the number of petechiae that develop are counted. Some petechiae are normal, but a marked increase in the number of petechiae is seen in scurvy. The platelet count, bleeding time, PT, and PTT are all generally *normal.*

Treatment is **oral vitamin C supplements** and **dietary counseling**. Symptoms usually start to improve within a week.

More High-Yield Facts

Niacin deficiency (vitamin **B3** deficiency, also called **pellagra**) causes the 4 "Ds": diarrhea, dermatitis, and dementia, and death (without treatment).

Vitamin B6 deficiency (**pyridoxine** deficiency) classically occurs in the setting of prolonged **isoniazid** therapy (e.g., tuberculosis therapy). Consider prophylactic supplements, especially in younger persons. Classic findings are **peripheral neuropathy** and cheilosis or stomatitis (i.e., mouth/lip fissures or irritation). Peripheral neuropathy can also occur with pyridoxine **toxicity** (the only B vitamin with known toxicity).

Vitamin A deficiency can cause **scaly skin, dry eyes** (xerophthalmia), and **night blindness**. It is the only **teratogenic** vitamin.

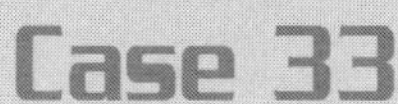

Internal Medicine

History

A 27-year-old man comes to your office because of recurrent episodes of chest pain for the last few weeks. The episodes last for several minutes, and the patient describes the pain as a sharp and burning, located under the sternum. The pain has occurred at least once per day for the past few weeks, but the patient has had previous attacks that were less frequent and severe. The pain often comes on at night when he is trying to fall asleep and is frequently associated with burping.

Past medical history is unremarkable, and the patient takes no regular medications. He smokes roughly 1 pack of cigarettes per day and has recently been drinking a lot of coffee at work due to an upcoming deadline and longer work hours. He doesn't normally drink alcohol very often, but mentions that he has been having a few drinks at night after work to unwind from the stress. Family history is noncontributory.

Exam

T: 98.7°F BP: 124/80 RR: 12/min. P: 66/min.

The patient is overweight, but in no acute distress. Head, neck, and chest exams are unremarkable. Abdominal exam reveals mild tenderness to deep palpation in the epigastric region, but no other abnormalities. The stool is negative for occult blood. The rest of the exam is normal.

Tests

Hemoglobin: 15 mg/dL (normal 14–18)
White blood cell count: 6900/μL (normal 4500–11,000)
Platelet count: 270,000/μL (normal 150,000–400,000)
Peripheral smear: within normal limits
AST: 14 u/L (normal 7–27)
EKG: normal sinus rhythm; no abnormalities

Condition Gastroesophageal reflux disease (GERD)

Pathophysiology

Inappropriate relaxation of the lower esophageal sphincter (LES) is thought to allow gastric contents to reflux into the esophagus, which causes irritation and symptoms. GERD is thought to occur in up to **40%** of adults on a **monthly** basis and close to **10%** on a **daily** basis.

GERD can lead to **asthma, aspiration** and **pneumonitis, GI bleeding, Barrett's esophagus/metaplasia** (a change from normal **squamous** epithelium to **intestinal columnar** epithelium with **goblet cells**), **esophageal stricture,** and **esophageal carcinoma**.

Diagnosis & Treatment

Symptoms include "**heartburn**" (retrosternal burning pain), abdominal discomfort, atypical **chest pain, burping, regurgitation** (reflux of gastric contents into the mouth), and **dysphagia** (classically described as food "sticking"). Chronic **cough, asthma, and hoarseness** are atypical presentations. Symptoms typically occur at **night,** when the patient **lays flat** to go to sleep.

Physical exam classically reveals **epigastric tenderness**. The diagnosis is often made presumptively in the setting of typical symptoms. In atypical cases or those with worrisome symptoms (e.g., weight loss, dysphagia), evaluation with **upper endoscopy** or an **upper GI series** is indicated. The gold standard for diagnosis is **24-hour esophageal pH monitoring**.

For the boards, treatment begins with **conservative measures** to improve LES tone and reduce esophageal irritation, including **cessation of smoking, caffeine, chocolate, alcohol abuse, and fatty and spicy foods**. **Weight loss** is also advised. Anticholinergic drugs and calcium channel blockers should be *stopped* if possible. The patient should be instructed to **elevate the head of the bed by several inches** and **avoid eating within 3 hours of bedtime**. If these measures fail, drug therapy with **antacids, H2-blockers,** or **proton pump inhibitors** is given. **Pro-motility agents** (e.g., metoclopramide) may also improve symptoms. **Antireflux surgery** (e.g., Nissen fundoplication) is an option when medical therapy fails.

In patients with refractory symptoms, especially when long-term, endoscopy should be considered to rule out **Barrett's esophagus**. If found, **regular endoscopy** surveillance is indicated to detect **early malignant transformation**. The frequency depends on the severity of dysplasia, and the guidelines are still evolving, but at least once every 1–2 years.

More High-Yield Facts

GERD is often associated with a sliding-type **hiatal hernia**.

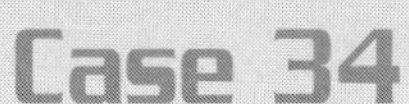

Internal Medicine

History

A 61-year-old woman has come to the emergency department because of gradually increasing shortness of breath, nausea, and fatigue that began a few weeks ago. She denies fever, chest pain, cough, and weight loss, but admits to fairly frequent leg cramps and "itchy skin." The patient knows little about her past medical history, but says she has had diabetes and high blood pressure for more than 20 years. She has been told that these conditions have affected her kidneys, but she is not on dialysis and denies any cardiac history. Her medications include metformin, insulin, and lisinopril. The patient does not smoke or drink alcohol. She states that she has missed the last several appointments to see her regular doctor, but claims to be compliant with her medications.

Exam

T: 98.6°F BP: 154/92 RR: 20/min. P: 88/min.

The patient is moderately tachypneic and prefers to sit straight up to minimize her dyspnea. Scleral pallor is evident. Her skin is slightly yellowish-brown. Chest exam reveals rales bilaterally in the lower one-third of the lung fields. Cardiac exam is normal. Abdominal exam is unremarkable, and the stool is negative for occult blood. Extremity exam reveals 2+ symmetric pitting edema in the lower extremities and decreased vibratory sensation in both lower extremities below the mid-shin level.

Tests

Hemoglobin: 9 mg/dL (normal 12–16)
Mean corpuscular volume: 90 µm/cell (normal 80–100)
White blood cell (WBCs) count: 7400/µL (normal 4500–11,000)
Platelet count: 270,000/µL (normal 150,000–400,000)
Ferritin: 160 µg/L (normal 20–200)
Sodium: 135 meq/L (normal 135–145)
Potassium: 5.8 meq/L (normal 3.5–5)
CO_2 content: 16 meq/L (normal 24–30)
Creatinine: 4.2 mg/dL
BUN: 48 mg/dL (normal 8–25)
Calcium: 8 mg/dL (normal 8.5–10.5)
Phosphorus: 5.7 mg/dL (normal 3–4.5)
Albumin: 3.6 mg/dL (normal 3.5–5)
EKG: normal sinus rhythm
Chest x-ray: normal-size cardiac silhouette and pulmonary edema
Urinalysis: 3± proteinuria; negative for glucose, bilirubin, and WBCs; prominent, broad, and waxy casts noted

Condition End-stage renal disease (ESRD)

Pathophysiology

The number one and two causes of ESRD are **diabetes mellitus** and **hypertension,** respectively, which account for well over half of cases. Other causes include **glomerulonephritis, collagen vascular diseases** (especially lupus), **polycystic kidney disease,** and **malignancy** (classic example is multiple myeloma).

Multiple derangements occur when the kidneys fail, including **electrolyte and acid-base disturbances, azotemia** (which can lead to neurologic, hematologic, dermatologic, cardiovascular, gastrointestinal, and immune system dysfunction), failure of **erythropoietin** secretion, and decreased **vitamin D** synthesis.

Diagnosis & Treatment

Common symptoms include **fatigue,** trouble thinking or concentrating, **shortness of breath** (from acidosis and volume overload), **muscle twitching** or **cramps, anorexia, nausea** and **vomiting, skin discoloration,** and **pruritus**.

Signs of ESRD include **anemia, muscle twitching, peripheral neuropathy** (can be from ESRD or coexisting diabetes), **hypertension, volume overload** (e.g., pulmonary congestion with rales, lower extremity edema), and **yellowish-brown skin discoloration (uremic "frost").** Uremic **pericarditis** may be present and can lead to a friction rub. Labs reveal **elevated BUN and creatinine, hyperkalemia, metabolic acidosis** (decreased CO_2 content), **hypocalcemia, hyperphosphatemia,** normochromic normocytic anemia, and **broad, waxy casts** on urinalysis. **Proteinuria** may also be seen, especially in cases due to diabetic nephropathy. The classic EKG in renal failure shows changes of hyperkalemia. X-rays may reveal **osteomalacia** (renal osteodystrophy) and pulmonary edema.

ESRD is irreversible, and the mainstay of treatment is **hemodialysis** while awaiting **renal transplant**. Dietary phosphate and potassium restrictions are advised, though often difficult to follow. **Erythropoietin** can be given to treat anemia. **Phosphate binders,** such as calcium carbonate, are also traditionally given, along with **vitamin D supplements** to lessen bone resorption. However, recent data suggest that these products may result in calcium overload and have made their use more controversial.

More High-Yield Facts

Put all **diabetic patients** on an **ACE-inhibitor** to slow progression of diabetic nephropathy to ESRD.

Case 35

Internal Medicine

History

A 26-year-old woman seeks medical advice for fatigue and a skin rash on her face, both of which have been steadily getting worse over the last few weeks. The patient denies recent sick contacts, fever, and vaginal discharge. A colleague in your office has seen the patient before for a large, painless oral ulcer of unknown etiology that resolved with conservative treatment. The patient takes no regular medications and has no chronic medical problems. She does not smoke, drink alcohol, or use illicit drugs. The patient is sexually active and has had multiple partners in the past year.

Exam

T: 99.4°F BP: 124/82 RR: 14/min. P: 78/min.

The patient is healthy appearing and in no acute distress. An erythematous, scaly rash is evident on her cheek and in the upper eyelid region (see figure). The skin is somewhat indurated in the affected area. Mild scleral pallor is present. The chest, abdomen, pelvic, extremity, and neurologic exams are normal. The stool is negative for occult blood.

Tests

Hemoglobin: 10 mg/dL (normal 12–16)
Mean corpuscular volume: 88/μL (normal 80–100)
White blood cell count: 5400/μL (normal 4500–11,000)
Platelet count: 70,000/μL (normal 150,000–400,000)
Ferritin: 280 μg/L (normal 20–200)
Creatinine: 1.1 mg/dL (normal 0.6–1.5)
Urinalysis: 2+ proteinuria; negative for glucose, bacteria, and bilirubin; granular casts noted
Erythrocyte sedimentation rate: 58 mm/hr (normal 0–20)
Antinuclear antibody (ANA): positive to a dilution of 1:512 (normal < 1:4)
HIV test: negative
VDRL syphilis test: negative

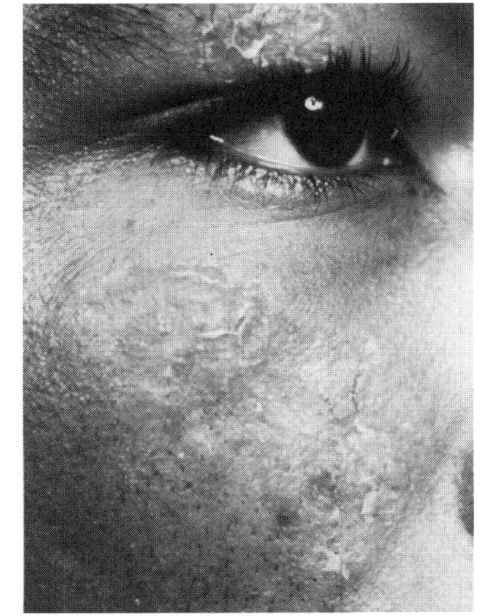

From David-Bajar KM. In Fitzpatrick JE, Aeling JL (eds): Dermatology Secrets, 2nd ed. Philadelphia, Hanley & Belfus, Inc., 2001, pp 155–162; with permission.

Condition

Systemic lupus erythematosus (SLE)

The photo shows a fairly typical appearance of a discoid lupus rash.

Pathophysiology

SLE is an **autoimmune** disorder most commonly seen in **reproductive-age females** and it is more common in **blacks** than whites. The immune system derangements can affect nearly every organ system. Death can occur secondary to complications from renal failure, hemorrhage, or infection (usually due to immunosuppression), but 10-year survival is at least **85%**.

Diagnosis & Treatment

A malar or discoid **skin rash, arthritis, fatigue,** and/or **fever** are the classic presenting complaints for SLE. Many other symptoms are also possible, however, ranging from psychosis to alopecia and mouth sores (ulcers).

SLE findings vary, but are broken down into 11 categories (four must be present to technically make a diagnosis, though not necessarily at the same time). **Malar rash** ("butterfly" rash over the cheeks and bridge of the nose), discoid rash, **photosensitivity, oral ulcers,** inflammatory-type **arthritis,** and **serositis** (e.g., **pleuritis** or **pericarditis**) are six of the categories. The other five are **renal abnormalities** (e.g., **proteinuria** or **casts**), **neurologic** abnormalities (e.g., **seizures, psychosis, major depression**), **hematologic** abnormalities (**anemia, leukopenia, thrombocytopenia**), **immunologic** abnormalities (positive **anti-DNA** or **anti-Smith** antibodies or a **false-positive VDRL/RPR** syphilis test), and a **positive ANA** titer. **Alopecia,** weight loss, myalgias, Raynaud's phenomenon, personality changes, myocarditis, adenopathy, and hepatosplenomegaly are other possible findings. The **lupus anticoagulant** may be present; it can result in **recurrent venous thrombosis** and **recurrent miscarriages,** though the **partial thromboplastin time** is generally **prolonged**.

For practical purposes, the **screening** test for SLE is the ANA antibody titer, and the **confirmatory** test is the anti-Smith antibody titer. Treatment consists of **anti-inflammatory drugs, hydroxychloroquine,** and **corticosteroids**. Immunosuppressants such as methotrexate or cyclophosphamide may be needed in severe cases. The course is variable, ranging from relentless progression to occasional mild symptom flares. Prognosis is often related to the degree of **renal involvement**.

More High-Yield Facts

Drug-induced lupus is classically due to **hydralazine, procainamide,** or **isoniazid**.

Case 36

Internal Medicine

History

A 78-year-old woman with known Alzheimer's dementia is brought to the hospital by her daughter for refusal to eat, increasing confusion, and lethargy over the last few days. The patient is unable to answer questions. Her daughter indicates that she has moderately severe cognitive impairment at baseline and also has hypertension, chronic lower leg edema, and arthritis. The patient's only medications are furosemide and acetaminophen.

Exam

T: 98.4°F BP: 104/66 RR: 20/min. P: 112/min.

The patient is dyspneic and incoherent. Her mucous membranes are extremely dry, and marked skin tenting is present. Her chest is clear to auscultation. Cardiac exam reveals tachycardia with no murmurs. Abdominal and extremity examinations are unremarkable.

Tests

Hemoglobin: 17 mg/dL (normal 12–16)
White blood cell count: 8400/μL (normal 4500–11,000)
Platelet count: 340,000/μL (normal 150,000–400,000)
Sodium: 158 meq/L (normal 135–145)
Potassium: 3.6 meq/L (normal 3.5–5)
CO_2: 19 meq/L (normal 24–30)
Creatinine: 1.7 mg/dL (normal 0.6–1.5)
BUN: 60 mg/dL (normal 8–25)
Urinalysis: specific gravity 1.030; negative for protein, glucose, and bacteria

Condition Hypernatremia, secondary to marked dehydration

Pathophysiology

Most cases of hypernatremia are seen in the setting of **dehydration,** which may be secondary to **inadequate fluid intake, diuretics, diabetes insipidus, diarrhea,** and **renal disease**. Misuse of IV fluids can result in **iatrogenic** cases.

Diagnosis & Treatment

The main symptoms of hypernatremia are **neurologic,** and include **mental status changes, confusion,** and **lethargy**. Physical findings may include **hyperreflexia** or **seizures** in severe cases. Findings of dehydration (e.g., dry mucous membranes, skin tenting, BUN:creatinine ratio > 15:1, hypotension, tachycardia, high urine specific gravity) are usually present.

The diagnosis is made with laboratory testing, which reveals an **elevated sodium** level. Other electrolyte abnormalities may be present, such as **acidosis** related to severe dehydration and poor tissue perfusion and **azotemia** secondary to inadequate renal perfusion.

Treatment is generally **normal saline** to correct dehydration. The sodium level will return to normal on its own with correction of the dehydration in most cases. Most patients have a **total body deficit of sodium,** even though the level is high. In most cases, the initial use of ½ normal saline or other less concentrated forms of saline is *inappropriate,* though these may be indicated once the dehydration is corrected. The **underlying cause** must also be addressed. For example, the patient in the current example may need a skilled nursing facility and should have her furosemide held if she refuses to eat or drink appropriately. **Elder abuse** must also be considered in this particular case.

More High-Yield Facts

Furosemide/loop diuretics cause dehydration much more often than thiazide diuretics, as thiazides are often *self-limiting* in the amount of diuresis they can cause. Once a patient becomes mildly dehydrated, thiazides lose their ability to cause diuresis, while loop diuretics will generally *continue to cause diuresis* in this setting.

As with all electrolyte disturbances, *avoid* immediate rapid correction. **Gradual, conservative correction** of electrolyte disturbances is almost always preferred.

Case 37

Internal Medicine

History

A 68-year-old man comes into the office for a "flu shot." He says his wife made him come in because he hasn't seen a doctor in 15 years, and she thinks he should get a flu shot this year, because he got a "bad case of the flu" the previous winter. The man has no complaints and says he has been "blessed with excellent health." His past medical history is significant only for arthritis, for which the patient takes acetaminophen sporadically. The patient is monogamous and does not smoke or drink alcohol. His family history is noncontributory. He is a retired businessman and travels only within the United States.

Exam

T: 98.7°F BP: 136/84 RR: 12/min. P: 72/min.

The patient is healthy appearing and in no acute distress. Physical exam is normal. Specifically, the chest is clear, the stool tests negative for occult blood, and no rectal or prostate abnormalities are detected.

Given the patient's age and history, what vaccines would you recommend he receive?

Tests

Hemoglobin: 15 mg/dL (normal 14–18)
White blood cell count: 7000/μL (normal 4500–11,000)
Platelet count: 280,000/μL (normal 150,000–400,000)
Sodium: 138 meq/L (normal 135–145)
Potassium: 4.1 meq/L (normal 3.5–5)
Creatinine: 0.8 mg/dL (normal 0.6–1.5)
BUN: 9 mg/dL (normal 8–25)

Adult vaccine recommendations

Pathophysiology

Vaccination is an example of **primary prevention**. Preventative health is epidemiologically important and is fairly heavily tested on the boards.

Diagnosis & Treatment

The patient in this example should receive the influenza and pneumococcal vaccines as well as a tetanus/diphtheria booster. Vaccines and their indications for adults ≥ 18 years old are:

- **Influenza—all adults ≥ 50 years old;** residents of nursing homes or other facilities for patients with chronic medical conditions; those with chronic cardiovascular or pulmonary disorders (including **asthma**), chronic metabolic disorders (including **diabetes**), renal dysfunction, or hemoglobinopathies; and those who are immunosuppressed for any reason. **Contraindicated** if person has an **anaphylactic allergy to eggs**.
- **Tetanus/diphtheria (Td)—all adults every 10 years**. For all but clean, minor wounds, give Td booster if more than **5 years** since last dose.
- ***Pneumococcus*—all adults ≥ 65 years old;** those with chronic cardiovascular or pulmonary disorders, other immunosuppressive chronic conditions (including diabetes, alcoholism, chronic liver disorders, splenic dysfunction/asplenia, multiple myeloma, and renal failure). Those vaccinated prior to age 65 should receive a **second dose** at age 65 if it has been more than 5 years since the first dose.
- **Hepatitis B**—those with occupational risk (e.g., blood/body fluid exposure), staff and residents in institutions, prisoners, hemodialysis patients, regular recipients of blood products, household contacts/sexual partners of those with hepatitis B, international travelers, IV drug users, homosexual men, and promiscuous heterosexuals. **Contraindicated** in those with an **anaphylactic yeast allergy**.
- **Hepatitis A**—those who travel to or work in high-risk countries, homosexual men, IV drug abusers, and those with chronic liver disease or clotting factor disorders. Also consider in frequent food handlers.

More High-Yield Facts

Always consider health maintenance/prevention in all patients! Attending to preventive health issues may be the best answer to a question about a patient with totally unrelated complaints.

In general, *avoid* vaccines during an acute febrile illness or if there is a history of previous severe reaction to a vaccine. Give basic vaccines to patients who request them (e.g., hepatitis A and B, influenza).

Case 38

Internal Medicine

History

A 62-year-old man is experiencing shortness of breath on exertion. He says his symptoms have come on gradually over the last week or so. The patient denies fever, cough, sick contact, chest pain, diaphoresis, and weight loss. His past medical history is fairly unremarkable, and he takes no regular medications. He smokes roughly a pack a day of cigarettes and drinks alcohol "occasionally." Family history is noncontributory

Exam

T: 98.9°F BP: 134/88 RR: 16/min. P: 82/min.

The patient is mildly overweight, but in no acute distress. Head, neck, and cardiac exams are unremarkable. Lung exam reveals dullness to percussion in the right base, with absent breath sounds, decreased egophony, and decreased tactile fremitus. The remaining lung fields are clear to auscultation. Abdominal, rectal, extremity, and neurologic exams are all unremarkable.

Tests

Hemoglobin: 15 mg/dL (normal 14–18)
White blood cell (WBC) count: 7700/μL (normal 4500–11,000)
Platelets: 290,000/μL (normal 150,000–400,000)
Urinalysis: negative for glucose, protein, bacteria, and WBCs
EKG: normal
Chest x-ray: see figure

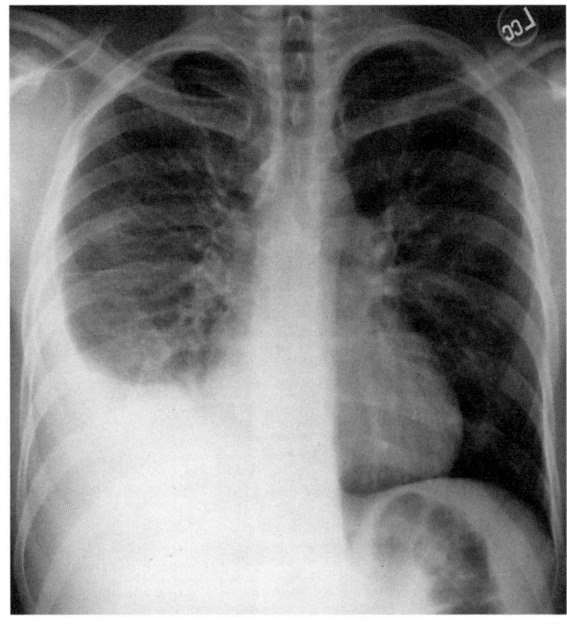

From Sahn SA, Heffner JE: Pulmonary Pearls II. Philadelphia, Hanley & Belfus, Inc., 1995, p 85; with permission.

Condition

Pleural effusion of unknown etiology

The chest x-ray shows a **right-sided pleural effusion** with a normal cardiac silhouette and no masses or infiltrates.

Pathophysiology

Pleural fluid can accumulate whenever there is excess pleural fluid formation or decreased fluid removal by the lymphatic system. Pleural fluid is generally characterized as exudative or transudative. **Exudative effusions** are due to **local factors** and are often (not always) **unilateral,** such as from infection, malignancy, some cases of pulmonary embolism (PE), pancreatitis, and collagen-vascular diseases. **Transudative effusions** are due to **systemic factors** and are often (not always) **bilateral,** such as from heart failure, cirrhosis, nephrotic syndrome, and some cases of PE.

Diagnosis & Treatment

The classic symptom of a pleural effusion is **shortness of breath**. Symptoms of the underlying disorder (e.g., fever and cough with pneumonia) are also usually present. Physical exam reveals **absent breath sounds, decreased egophony, decreased tactile fremitus,** and **dullness to percussion** in the region of the effusion.

In this example, the etiology of the effusion cannot be determined from the given information. In such cases, **thoracentesis** should be performed. Thoracentesis can also be performed for **symptom relief**. In cases of diagnostic uncertainty, pleural fluid should be analyzed for **glucose, amylase, LDH, total protein, cell count and differential, cytology, gram stain,** and **culture** (including tuberculosis and fungal cultures in at-risk patients). Pleural fluid is characterized as exudative when: the **pleural fluid protein:serum protein ratio > 0.5;** the **pleural fluid LDH:serum LDH ratio > 0.6;** or the pleural fluid LDH is more than two-thirds upper normal serum LDH. Transudative effusions are most often *benign* and typically require little further work-up.

In cases of effusion associated with pneumonia (parapneumonic effusion), thoracentesis should generally be performed to see if **tube thoracostomy** is needed. If pus, bacteria, low glucose (< 50 mg/dL), or low pH (< 7) is present in the fluid, a thoracostomy tube is generally advised to **prevent loculation** of the fluid, which can lead to empyema and the need for surgical decortication/drainage.

More High-Yield Facts

If the pleural fluid has a **high amylase level,** consider pancreatitis (usually a left-sided effusion), esophageal rupture, or malignancy. "**Milky**" pleural fluid with a **high triglyceride level** is due to a chylothorax (usually from injury to or malignant invasion of the thoracic duct).

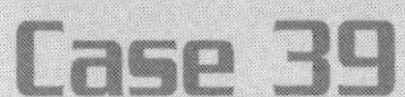

Case 39

Internal Medicine

History

A 36-year-old man visits the emergency department complaining of nausea, fatigue, and poor appetite that began 6 days ago. The patient denies sick contacts, cough, and weight loss, but mentions that his urine has become rather dark. Past medical history is unremarkable, and the patient does not take any regular medications. He admits to being promiscuous and is bisexual. The patient says he smokes cigarettes and marijuana and likes to drink alcohol "socially." He denies intravenous drug abuse.

Exam

T: 100.5°F BP: 130/84 RR: 14/min. P: 86/min.

The patient is thin and has scleral icterus. No adenopathy is appreciated. The chest exam is unremarkable. Abdominal exam reveals tender hepatomegaly, with a soft, smooth liver edge. Bowel sounds are normal, and no splenomegaly is detectable. The stool is negative for occult blood. Extremity exam reveals several small scabs on his right forearm, consistent with needle marks.

Tests

Hemoglobin: 15 mg/dL (normal 14–18)
White blood cell count: 5300/μL (normal 4500–11,000)
Platelets: 200,000/μL (normal 150,000–400,000)
AST: 584 u/L (normal 7–27)
ALT: 612 u/L (normal 1–21)
Bilirubin, total: 3.4 mg/dL (normal 0.1–1)
Bilirubin, direct: 1.6 mg/dL (normal 0–0.4)
Alkaline phosphatase: 45 u/L (normal 13–39)
Urinalysis: elevated urobilinogen; negative for glucose, protein, and bacteria
Hepatitis A IgM: negative
Hepatitis B surface antigen: positive
Hepatitis B surface IgM antibody: negative
Hepatitis B core IgM antibody: positive
Hepatitis B core IgG antibody: negative
Hepatitis B e antigen: positive
Hepatitis B e IgM antibody: negative
Hepatitis C IgM antibody: negative
Hepatitis D IgM antibody: negative

Condition Hepatitis B, acute

Pathophysiology

Acute viral hepatitis is most often due to one of the named hepatitis viruses (e.g., A through E). Other causes of infectious hepatitis (e.g., cytomegalovirus, Epstein-Barr virus) and noninfectious causes (e.g., alcoholic or drug-induced hepatitis, autoimmune hepatitis) must also be considered in the appropriate setting. Hepatitis **A and E** cause **acute hepatitis only,** while hepatitis **B, C and D** can cause **chronic hepatitis,** which can lead to **cirrhosis** and **hepatocellular carcinoma**. Hepatitis D can *only* occur in the setting of **coexisting hepatitis B** infection.

Diagnosis & Treatment

Classic acute hepatitis symptoms vary from mild to fulminant and include **anorexia, nausea, vomiting, lethargy, dark-colored urine, jaundice,** and **abdominal discomfort or pain**. The viral causes of acute hepatitis can all present in a similar fashion, and can generally only be distinguished by **serology**. Hepatitis A (common) and E (rare) are transmitted via the **fecal-oral route,** so are most likely in those who are not promiscuous, don't use IV drugs, and haven't received blood transfusions. The presence of these risk factors, however, is a warning sign for possible hepatitis B, C, or D, which is transmitted **parenterally**. Donated blood is screened for hepatitis.

Exam may reveal **jaundice, low-grade fever,** and **tender hepatomegaly**. The urine is often dark due to the presence of bilirubin products (remember, only **direct bilirubin** is filtered into the urine). **Hepatic transaminases** and **bilirubin** (direct and indirect) are usually elevated when acute symptoms occur. **Alkaline phosphatase** is usually only *mildly elevated,* and the **white blood cell** count is usually *normal.*

Hepatitis is generally diagnosed by the presence of a positive **IgM antibody titer** (IgG = old infection/exposure or chronicity) to a specific hepatitis virus. Hepatitis B serology is more tricky, and is commonly asked about on the boards. The **hepatitis B surface antigen (HBsAg)** indicates **active infection,** and its disappearance coincides with the appearance of **hepatitis B surface IgM antibody (HBsAb),** indicating **recovery**. HBsAg stays positive and HBsAb negative with chronic hepatitis B. The **hepatitis B core IgM antibody (HBcAb)** is the best marker for **acute infection** and may be the only positive marker acutely (this occurs during the so-called "**window period**"). **Hepatitis e antigen** is a marker for increased infectivity. Treatment is supportive acutely.

More High-Yield Facts

Hepatitis B vaccination causes a **positive HBsAb** with a **negative HBcAb,** while prior exposure/resolved infection causes **both to be positive**.

Case 40

Internal Medicine

History

A 62-year-old woman with known metastatic pancreatic cancer diagnosed 3 months ago wishes to discuss her care. She has decided that she no longer wants to pursue chemotherapy or other care for her cancer. The patient says she is comfortable with her condition and prognosis, which are dismal due to extensive metastasis. She wishes only to be comfortable and asks for your help "when the end comes." The patient says she wants no resuscitative measures performed—specifically, no CPR or "breathing machines." Her only wish is to avoid pain. The woman is calm, coherent, oriented, and appropriate. She denies all symptoms of depression and does not seem clinically depressed.

Three weeks later, you are called to the emergency department to see the patient.

Exam

T: 104.5°F   BP: 90/54   RR: 24/min.   P: 126/min.

The patient is tachypneic, delirious, and toxic appearing. You feel that the woman will not survive without aggressive medical management, including intubation and mechanical ventilation. The patient's husband is with her, and he demands to know what you plan to do to keep her alive. When you explain your meeting with her 3 weeks prior, the husband becomes upset and threatens to sue if immediate aggressive medical management is not performed. What is the best course of action in this situation?

Tests

None

Issue "Do not resuscitate" (DNR) order and end-of-life decisions

Pathophysiology

All patients must ultimately decide what treatments they will undergo. While some patients prefer to leave the decisions in the hands of their physicians, others have strong opinions of their own. The fact is that **any competent adult patient can refuse any medical intervention**. Even simple measures, such as antibiotics for uncomplicated community-acquired pneumonia, can be declined.

Diagnosis & Treatment

Give all competent adults a chance to decide their own treatment after explaining the risks and benefits of, and the alternatives to, the treatment you think is best. A "mini" mental status exam and brief conversation with a patient are generally enough to determine competence. If there is any difficulty in ascertaining competence, a **psychiatric consultation** is appropriate. Watch for **depression** in these situations, which is a form of "incompetence" when it comes to end-of-life decisions. Do not respect a patient's wish to die if he or she is depressed; treat the depression first!

A competent patient makes his or her own decisions. If a family member disagrees with the patient's decision, this is *not* relevant. The patient's wishes take precedence. However, family members/loved ones should be **treated with compassion and respect**. The boards may ask you what you would say to angry, dissenting family member. **Be kind, do not judge, sit down and discuss the issues and patient's wishes, and ask about their concerns**. The threat of a lawsuit should never deter you on the boards (forget the real world . . .). In difficult cases, consider involving the **hospital ethics committee** and, as a last resort, the courts.

If a patient is incompetent or unable to communicate, healthcare decisions are usually left up to the **closest relative**. This person should be instructed to make decisions **based on what the patient would have wanted** (*not* what the relative wants). When possible, **healthcare power of attorney** should be obtained for healthcare decisions, to help prevent family conflicts and give the legal right of decision-making to one specific person.

More High-Yield Facts

Don't be afraid to discuss end-of-life issues with patients prior to the acute situation. Opening up a discussion will *not* cause a patient to commit suicide or choose a "DNR" status.

For boards purposes, **passive euthanasia** (i.e., allowing disease to cause death, or withdrawing care) is okay, but **active euthanasia** (i.e., directly causing a patient to die to relieve suffering) is not.

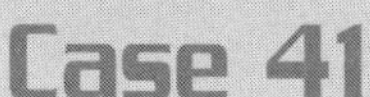

Case 41

Internal Medicine

History

A 57-year-old man comes into your office complaining of increasing weakness, poor appetite, and increasing abdominal distension that is making it harder to breathe. He also mentions dark-colored urine and yellow discoloration of his eyes. The patient is a known alcoholic who you haven't seen in a few years. He says he has been hospitalized twice in the last 3 months for vomiting blood, and was told he had "big veins" around his stomach. The patient says he has been unable to cut down on his drinking. Past medical history is only notable for alcoholism for the past 20 years and complications from it, including gastritis, alcoholic hepatitis, and aspiration pneumonia. The patient takes no medications.

Exam

T: 98.6°F BP: 138/86 RR: 18/min. P: 86/min.

The patient is mildly tachypneic, but in no acute distress. Scleral pallor and icterus as well as bilateral parotid gland enlargement are noted. He has a paucity of body hair. Chest exam is notable for gynecomastia and multiple, small but prominent vessels on the chest wall and neck; smaller vessels radiate out from the central vessel like the legs of a spider. Abdominal exam reveals marked abdominal protruberance, bulging flanks, a positive fluid wave, and visibly enlarged abdominal wall veins. Bowel sounds are normal. His liver is enlarged and nontender, with a hard, nodular consistency on palpation. His spleen is palpable below the left costal margin. Rectal exam reveals stool that is weakly positive for occult blood; the testicles are atrophic. Extremity exam demonstrates palmar erythema, muscular wasting, and 2+ pitting edema of the lower extremities.

Tests

Hemoglobin: 11 mg/dL (normal 14–18)
Mean corpuscular volume: 104 μm/cell
White blood cell count: 5300/μL (normal 4500–11,000)
Platelet count: 100,000/μL (normal 150,000–400,000)
Peripheral smear: macrocytosis, 2+ acanthocytes, 2+ target cells
AST: 86 u/L (normal 7–27)
ALT: 40 u/L (normal 1–21)
Bilirubin, total: 3.2 mg/dL (normal 0.1–1)
Bilirubin, direct: 1.4 mg/dL (normal 0–0.4)
Albumin: 2.4 mg/dL (normal 3.5–5)
Prothrombin time: 23 seconds (normal 10–15)

Cirrhosis

Pathophysiology

Cirrhosis is characterized by widespread liver **fibrosis** associated with attempts at repair resulting in **regenerative nodules**. It is considered **irreversible** and is usually due to **alcohol abuse** or **chronic viral hepatitis**. Other causes (e.g., hemochromatosis, Wilson's disease, cystic fibrosis, chronic biliary disease, alpha-1 antitrypsin deficiency) are less common. Cirrhosis causes **liver insufficiency** with resultant widespread metabolic and physiologic abnormalities. It is a common cause of death.

Diagnosis & Treatment

Symptoms of cirrhosis include **jaundice, anorexia, weakness, weight loss, malaise, dark-colored urine, edema, impotence,** and symptoms from complications of **portal hypertension** (e.g., ascites, hematemesis from variceal bleeding). Extensive ascites can cause **dyspnea**.

Exam classically reveals **parotid enlargement, jaundice, ascites** (e.g., positive fluid wave, bulging flanks, shifting dullness to percussion), **splenomegaly,** a **hard and nodular liver** that may be enlarged or shrunken (end-stage), **peripheral edema, muscle wasting,** and enlarged abdominal wall veins (**caput medusae**). Increased estrogen levels can lead to **spider angiomas** (the lesions on this patient's chest and neck, the classic locations), **decreased body hair, gynecomastia, palmar erythema,** and **testicular atrophy**. **Asterixis** and **encephalopathy** can also be seen.

Labs usually reveal some **elevation of all liver function tests,** especially **bilirubin**. **Low albumin, prolonged prothrombin time,** and a **macrocytic anemia** (may see target cells or acanthocytes on peripheral smear) are also often present. **Elevated ammonia levels** can result in encephalopathy. **Liver biopsy** confirms the diagnosis and may help determine the etiology in the rare cases with an unknown etiology.

Basic treatment includes **alcohol cessation,** a **salt and protein-restricted diet, diuretics,** and "as-needed" **paracentesis**. Encephalopathy is treated with **lactulose** and protein restriction to decrease serum ammonia. Severe portal hypertension may require a **portosystemic shunt,** either by the preferred **transjugular intrahepatic portosystemic shunt (TIPS)** procedure or by **surgical** shunt creation. Cirrhosis carries a poor prognosis, with roughly one-third of patients dying within a year. **Liver transplant** is the only cure.

More High-Yield Facts

Spontaneous bacterial peritonitis occurs in those with ascites and classically causes **fever** and an **increased neutrophil count** in the ascitic fluid. Treat with **antibiotics** to cover bowel flora.

Case 42

Internal Medicine

History

A 32-year-old Mediterranean woman has made an appointment because she is new in town and needs a new doctor. She has no complaints and is in good health. Her past medical history is significant for anemia, and she has been taking iron for the last 2 months. The patient says her prescription from her old doctor is about to run out, and she will need a refill. She does not smoke or drink alcohol.

Exam

T: 98.7°F BP: 118/76 RR: 12/min. P: 76/min.

The patient is thin and in no acute distress. Mild scleral pallor is noted. Chest, abdominal, rectal, and pelvic exams are unremarkable. No skin or extremity abnormalities are detected. Results of a neurologic exam are normal.

Tests

Hemoglobin: 10 mg/dL (normal 12–16)
Mean corpuscular volume: 72 μm/cell
White blood cell count: 7300/μL (normal 4500–11,000)
Platelet count: 300,000/μL (normal 150,000–400,000)
Iron level: 130 μg/dL (normal 50–150)
Ferritin level: 190 μg/L (normal 20–200)
Total iron-binding capacity: 270 μg/dL (normal 250–410)
Hemoglobin A_2: 5% (normal $< 3.5\%$)
Peripheral blood smear: see figure

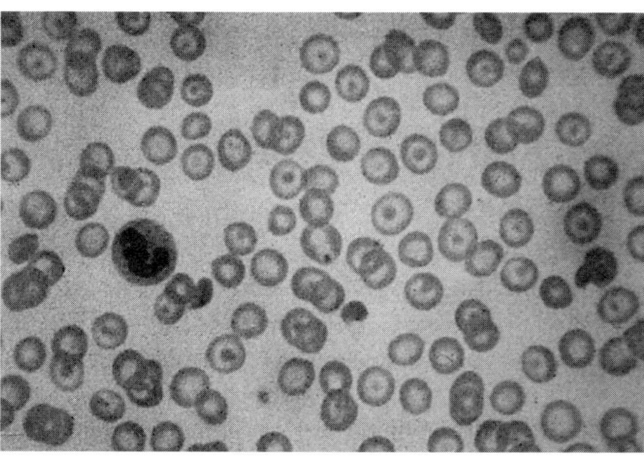

From Lukens J. In Lee GR, et al (eds): Wintrobe's Clinical Hematology, 10th ed. Philadelphia, Williams & Wilkins, 1999, pp 1405–1448; with permission.

Condition

Thalassemia (beta-thalassemia minor)

The peripheral smear reveals hypochromic red blood cells with many target cells (dark center portion in several RBCs).

Pathophysiology

Thalassemia is a heterogeneous group of genetic disorders that all result in **decreased or absent production** of specific **globin chains** present in normal hemoglobin. The clinical severity can range from in utero death to an absence of symptoms. Minor cases of thalassemia are important to recognize because they may cause a microcytic, hypochromic anemia that **can be confused with iron-deficiency anemia**. Thalassemia is most common in those of **African, Mediterranean, Middle Eastern,** and **Asian** descent.

There are four alpha-globin genes, and patients affected with clinically apparent alpha-thalassemia (at least two of four alpha genes deleted) have abnormalities **at birth** (and even in utero). There are only two beta-globin genes, and those affected with beta-thalassemia are usually not symptomatic until **after 4 or 5 months of age** due to the presence of fetal hemoglobin at birth.

Diagnosis & Treatment

Adult patients either have a known history of thalassemia or are asymptomatic (because moderate to severe cases will present in the pediatric age group). Asymptomatic adults have **microcytic, hypochromic red blood cells** and usually a **mild anemia** that is often incidentally discovered. However, **iron studies are normal** in those with thalassemia, distinguishing it from iron-deficiency anemia. On Step 2, the classic question about **beta-thalassemia minor** will mention either an **elevated hemoglobin A_2** or **elevated hemoglobin F,** both of which allow a presumptive diagnosis and are *not* seen with alpha-thalassemia minor.

The main reasons to confirm the diagnosis are to prevent the use of iron therapy (e.g., **patient education**), which can result in **iron overload** in these patients, and to consider the implications for **genetic counseling**. Education and counseling are the sole treatments for asymptomatic individuals.

More High-Yield Facts

Cooley's anemia is beta-thalassemia major (homozygous beta-thalassemia). These patients present in **infancy** and require repeated transfusions and **iron chelation**. Bone marrow transplant can be curative.

Deletion of all four alpha-globin genes causes in utero fetal death (**fetal hydrops**). Deletion of three alpha-globin genes causes **hemoglobin H disease,** which is somewhat similar clinically to beta-thalassemia major.

Case 43

Internal Medicine

History

A 37-year-old man is suffering from gnawing epigastric abdominal pain. He says he has had bouts of this pain occasionally for several years, but for the last 2 weeks it has become more frequent and intense. The pain often comes on 2 or 3 hours after a meal and is relieved by eating again or drinking milk. The patient has no significant past medical history and takes no medications. He smokes a pack of cigarettes per day, drinks several cups of coffee per day, and has 3–4 beers each night when he gets home from work.

Exam

T: 98.8°F BP: 128/84 RR: 14/min. P: 78/min.

The patient is mildly overweight, but in no acute distress. Head, neck, and chest exams are unremarkable. Epigastric tenderness is noted on abdominal exam, with no peritoneal signs and normal bowel sounds. No organomegaly is appreciated. Stool is negative for occult blood. No other abnormalities are noted.

Tests

Hemoglobin: 15 mg/dL (normal 14–18)
White blood cell count: 7500/μL (normal 4500–11,000)
Platelet count: 240,000/μL (normal 150,000–400,000)
AST: 10 u/L (normal 7–27)
Amylase: 58 u/L (normal 53–123)
Lipase: 12 u/L (normal 4- 24)
Upper GI series: see figure

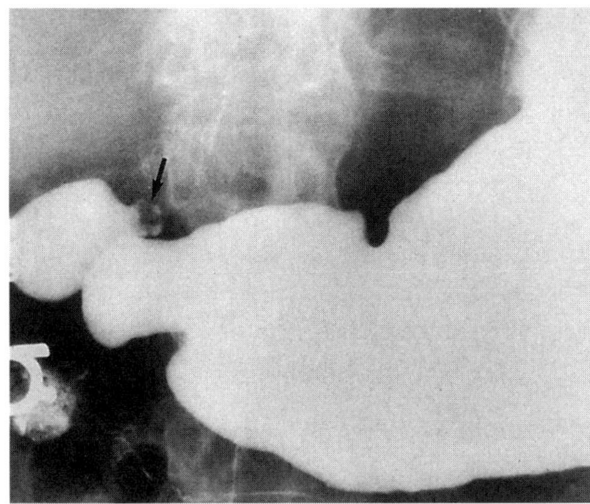

From Gastrointestinal imaging. In Daffner RH: Clinical Radiology: The Essentials. Philadelphia, Williams & Wilkins, 1999, pp 287–340; with permission.

Condition **Peptic ulcer disease (PUD)**

The x-ray shows the classic appearance of an ulcer crater (*arrow*), which is only partially filled with contrast.

Pathophysiology

Peptic ulcer disease is present when mucosal damage in the stomach or duodenum occurs due to an **imbalance** between gastric acid and mucosal protective factors. Though gastric acid is *required* for ulcer development, the amount of acid present may be **low, normal, or high** in those with PUD. The majority of cases of PUD (roughly 75%) occur in the **duodenum**. Risk factors for PUD include ***Helicobacter pylori*** infection (primarily duodenal ulcers), **NSAID use** (primarily gastric ulcers), and **smoking**. Coffee and alcohol use can delay healing or aggravate symptoms in some patients. **Zollinger-Ellison syndrome** is a gastrinoma that results in severe ulcers.

Diagnosis & Treatment

The classic symptom of PUD is **gnawing, burning or aching epigastric abdominal pain**. In cases of *duodenal* ulcer, the symptoms typically occur **2–3 hours after eating** and are **relieved by eating, drinking milk, or taking antacids**. *Gastric* ulcers are less related to food and may sometimes be **made worse by eating**. PUD can also present with **atypical chest pain**.

Physical exam reveals **epigastric tenderness**. The exam is otherwise unremarkable unless complications have occurred (e.g., hemorrhage, perforation, gastric outlet obstruction). The gold standard for diagnosis confirmation is **endoscopy,** which is more expensive, but also more sensitive, and allows biopsy to exclude malignancy with gastric ulcers and to test for *H. pylori*. An **upper GI barium series** is less expensive and has a lower risk of complications, but it is less sensitive.

Treatment includes **smoking cessation** and **moderation** in the use of alcohol, coffee, and any irritating (e.g., spicy or acidic) foods. In addition, **acid-reducing medications** (e.g., H2-blockers, proton-pump inhibitors) are given to allow ulcer healing. Adjunctive medications include **antacids** (for prompt relief of symptom flares) and **sucralfate** (mucosal protectant). NSAIDs should be *stopped,* especially with gastric ulcers. Testing for *H. pylori* can be done at the time of endoscopy or using **serology** or a breath test. Multiple drug regimens exist for *H. pylori* **eradication** (e.g., **proton-pump inhibitor plus two antibiotics,** such as clarithromycin and amoxicillin), if testing is positive, to aid healing and reduce recurrence rate. Surgery may be needed for complications (perforation, hemorrhage that can't be controlled endoscopically) or for medical therapy failure.

More High-Yield Facts

"Stress" ulcers are related to severe physical stress, such as burns (**Curling's ulcer**) or head trauma (**Cushing's ulcer**).

Case 44

Internal Medicine

History

A 57-year-old man complains of increasing shortness of breath over the last few months. He says he is used to being short of breath with physical exertion, but has started to become short of breath when performing basic daily activities. The patient denies fever, sick contacts, and weight loss. He says he has a chronic cough that is occasionally productive of whitish sputum, but he has not noticed any recent change in the frequency or character of his cough. He does not take any regular medications. He has smoked 1–2 packs of cigarettes per day for the past 35 years.

Exam

T: 98.8°F BP: 138/88 RR: 18/min. P: 88/min.

The patient is thin and mildly dyspneic. You notice that he seems to breathe through pursed lips and has a prolonged expiratory phase during quiet breathing. He has an increased anteroposterior chest diameter. Lung exam reveals no evidence of consolidation or focal abnormality; however, fairly diffuse mild end-expiratory wheezing is heard. Cardiac exam reveals somewhat faint heart sounds with no murmurs. Pulse oximetry on room air reveals an oxygen saturation of 88%.

Tests

Hemoglobin: 18 mg/dL (normal 14–18)
WBCs: 7100/μL (normal 4500–11,000)
Chest x-ray: see figure
EKG: normal sinus rhythm with evidence of right ventricular hypertrophy
Pulmonary function tests (PFTs)
  Forced vital capacity (FVC): 98% of predicted
  Forced expiratory volume in first second (FEV_1)/FVC: 45%

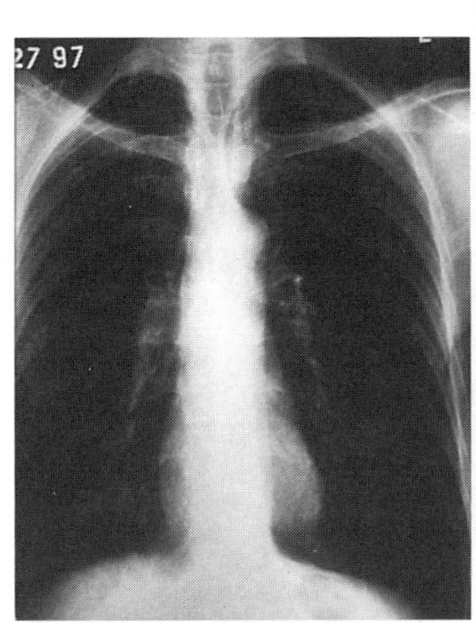

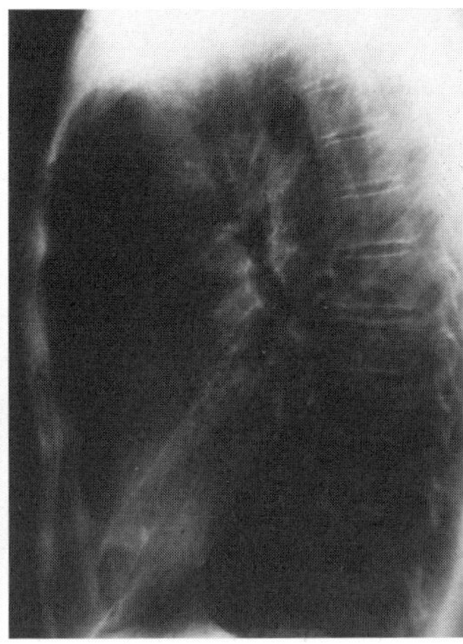

From Pulmonary imaging. In Daffner RH: Clinical Radiology: The Essentials. Philadelphia, Williams & Wilkins, 1999, pp 73–181; with permission.

Condition Chronic obstructive pulmonary disease (COPD)

The x-ray shows pulmonary hyperinflation, flattening of the diaphragm, and increased retrosternal clear space on the lateral view—all classic for emphysema.

Pathophysiology

The term COPD is used to describe the airway obstruction associated with **chronic bronchitis** and/or **emphysema,** which frequently coexist. Asthma is considered a separate disorder, though it also results in obstructive airway physiology. The cause of COPD is almost always **smoking**. **Alpha-1 antitrypsin deficiency** is a rare autosomal recessive cause of emphysema in young patients with no smoking history. Histologically, emphysema results in destruction of the alveolar walls and enlarged distal air spaces, **reducing the surface area available for gas exchange**. COPD is a common cause of death and can lead to right heart hypertrophy/failure (**cor pulmonale**).

Diagnosis & Treatment

The primary symptom of COPD is **shortness of breath**. Most patients also have a **chronic cough** and **increased mucus/sputum production**. Patients generally have at least a **10–15 pack-year smoking history**.

Exam may reveal **pursed lip breathing, increased anteroposterior chest diameter ("barrel chest"), prolonged expiratory phase** of respiration, **end-expiratory wheezing, use of accessory muscles of respiration, hyperresonance to percussion** and hypoxemia, cyanosis, and signs of right heart failure in advanced cases. Pulse oximetry or arterial blood gases may reveal **hypoxia** and/or **hypercapnia**. PFTs are generally used to confirm the diagnosis. PFTs reveal a **near-normal FVC** in most cases, but an abnormally **decreased FEV_1:FVC ratio (< 75%)**. The residual volume is generally *increased* in COPD.

In all cases, **smoking cessation** is desired, with drugs (nicotine, buproprion) and behavioral interventions used if needed. For mild COPD, treatment with an "as-needed" **anticholinergic** (generally ipratropium, which reduces airway secretions) and/or a **beta-2 agonist metered-dose inhaler** is useful. Patients with an oxygen saturation < 88% (pulse oximetry) or PaO2 < 55 mmHg (arterial blood gas) should be given home **oxygen, a treatment that has been shown to reduce mortality**. Give pneumococcal and annual influenza vaccines in all cases. COPD "**exacerbations**" are treated with oxygen and ipratropium/beta-2 agonists. Reserve **antibiotics** (e.g., amoxicillin, erythromycin) for those with **fever** or a **changed cough** (e.g., change in color or amount of sputum).

More High-Yield Facts

Empiric corticosteroid treatment is widely used, but largely unproven.

Case 45

Internal Medicine

History

A 62-year-old man with known lung cancer diagnosed 1 month ago is brought to the emergency department by his wife because of confusion that has been worsening over the past 4 days. The wife says that her husband doesn't seem to know where he is and has also become increasingly lethargic over the past 2 weeks. She states that he was mentally normal until 4–5 days ago. The patient has been taking morphine for pain control over the last month and has not increased his dosage. He takes no other medications. The wife denies fever or other symptoms.

Exam

T: 98.7°F BP: 138/88 RR: 14/min. P: 78/min.

The patient is disoriented to time and place and is unable to answer questions appropriately. He is non-toxic appearing and in no acute distress. Head, neck, chest, abdomen, and extremity exams are normal. No focal neurologic deficits are appreciated.

Tests

Hemoglobin: 14 mg/dL (normal 14–18)
White blood cell count: 7000/μL (normal 4500–11,000)
Creatinine: 0.5 mg/dL (normal 0.6–1.5)
BUN: 6 mg/dL (normal 8–25)
Fasting glucose: 90 mg/dL (normal 70–110)
Sodium: 122 meq/L (normal 135–145)
Potassium: 3.5 meq/L (normal 3.5–5)
Serum osmolality: 250 mOsm kg (normal 280–295)
Urine osmolality: 600 mOsm/kg
Urine sodium: 34 mmol/L
Chest x-ray: see figure

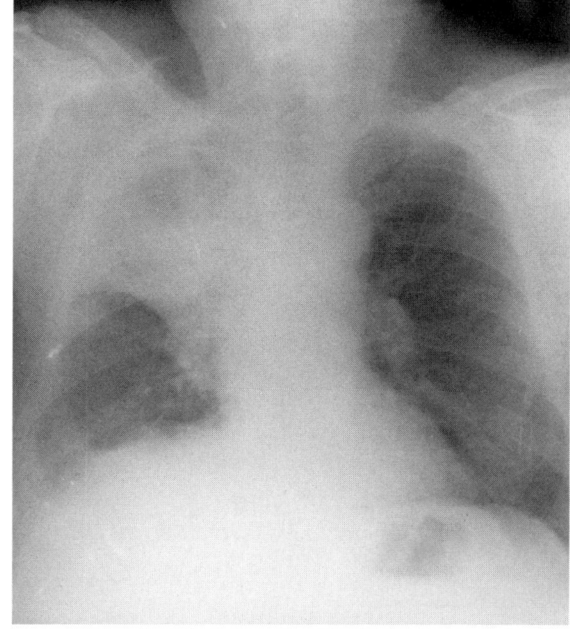

From Sahn SA, Heffner JE: Pulmonary Pearls II. Philadelphia, Hanley & Belfus, Inc., 1995, p 18; with permission.

Condition Syndrome of inappropriate antidiuretic hormone secretion (SIADH)

The chest x-ray reveals a right upper lobe mass.

Pathophysiology

Antidiuretic hormone (ADH) is secreted by the **posterior pituitar**y and causes **retention of free water** by the kidney and more concentrated urine. SIADH occurs if ADH is secreted without an appropriate physiologic stimulus (i.e., ADH is secreted "inappropriately"). There are several known causes of SIADH, including **malignancy** (classically, **small cell lung cancer**), **pulmonary diseases** (e.g., tuberculosis, pneumonia), **drugs** (e.g., narcotics, antineoplastics, oxytocin, carbamazepine), **hypothyroidism,** and **central nervous system disorders** (e.g., intracranial hemorrhage, meningitis). **Pain** and **nausea** also stimulate ADH release. SIADH can results in a vicious cycle of worsening hyponatremia.

Diagnosis & Treatment

Patients have symptoms of hyponatremia, such as **altered mental status** (e.g., confusion, irritability), **lethargy, weakness,** and possibly **seizures** or **coma** in severe cases. Risk factors for SIADH are generally present.

Exam reveals a **normal volume status:** this is important in the work-up of hyponatremia, as hyper- or hypovolemia should make you think of causes other than SIADH. **Hyponatremia** is present, and **most other serum lab values are low/below the normal range** (classic is low uric acid, creatinine, BUN, and albumin). **Serum osmolality** can be calculated

$$2(\text{sodium}) + \text{glucose}/18 + \text{BUN}/2.8$$

or measured directly and will be **low**. The urine osmolality will be **higher than the serum osmolality,** which is "inappropriate," as the body should be trying to dilute the urine to get rid of excess free water, not concentrating the urine. The **urine sodium concentration** is generally **> 20 mmol/L** (another marker for increased urine concentration).

Initial management is **water restriction** (< 1 L/day) and treating any reversible causes of SIADH (e.g., stop causative medications). If this fails, small amounts of normal saline plus loop diuretics (or hypertonic saline) can be given to **slowly correct hyponatremia over at least 24 hours,** as going faster may cause permanent **brainstem damage** (central pontine myelinolysis). **Demeclocycline** can be used in refractory chronic cases to cause renal diabetes insipidus.

More High-Yield Facts

Though often not needed, measuring serum ADH levels can confirm SIADH. ADH is *present* in SIADH, but generally *undetectable* with other causes of hyponatremia.

Case 46

Internal Medicine

History

A 19-year-old man presents to the emergency department with nausea, vomiting, and mild abdominal pain that began fairly suddenly several hours ago. Fatigue and frequent urination began 2–3 weeks ago and have become progressively worse. The patient has also noticed increased appetite and thirst, but thinks he may be losing weight. He has no significant past medical history and takes no medications. He is sexually active with his girlfriend of 2 years and uses condoms regularly. The patient does not smoke, drink alcohol, or use illicit drugs.

Exam

T: 98.3°F BP: 116/74 RR: 20/min. P: 98/min.

The patient is thin and tachypneic, taking rapid deep breaths. You note a peculiar fruity odor on his breath. The mucous membranes are quite dry. No adenopathy is appreciated. The chest exam is unremarkable, and the patient has mild diffuse abdominal tenderness to palpation. Extremity and neurologic exams are unremarkable.

Tests

Hemoglobin: 17 mg/dL (normal 14–18)
White blood cell count: 10,600/μL (normal 4500–11,000)
Platelets: 340,000/μL (normal 150,000–400,000)
Sodium: 133 meq/L (normal 135–145)
Potassium: 5.5 meq/L (normal 3.5–5)
CO_2: 8 meq/L (normal 24–30 meq/L)
Creatinine: 1.0 mg/dL (normal 0.6–1.5)
BUN: 25 mg/dL (normal 8–25)
Glucose: 590 mg/dL (normal random: < 200)
Arterial blood gas pH: 7.16 (normal 7.35–7.45)
Serum ketones: positive
Urinalysis: 2+ ketones, 4+ glucose; negative for protein and bacteria

Condition Diabetes mellitus type I (DM I)

The present patient has DM I of new onset, with ketoacidosis.

Pathophysiology

DM I accounts for roughly 10% of cases of DM. Affected persons have **decreased insulin secretion**. An **immunologic process** is the suspected cause, as **antibodies** against pancreatic islet cells are usually present at the time of initial diagnosis. Histopathology reveals **insulitis,** or active inflammation that causes loss of pancreatic beta cells. Certain **HLA types** (e.g., DR3 and DR4) increase the risk of DM I. Most cases present **prior to age 30**. The twin concurrence rate is roughly **50%** in DM I (versus > 90% in DM II). Those with DM I need exogenous insulin and *do not respond* to medications that increase endogenous insulin secretion (e.g., sulfonylureas).

Long-term, DM commonly causes **end-stage renal disease, blindness, atherosclerosis, sensory** and **autonomic neuropathy,** and an **increased risk of infections**. Aggressive treatment can lead to **hypoglycemia,** which is sometimes fatal and is now thought to have long-term neurologic effects.

Diagnosis & Treatment

Initial symptoms include **lethargy/fatigue, polyuria, polydipsia, polyphagia,** and **weight loss**. Patients may present with diabetic ketoacidosis (DKA), which can cause **nausea, vomiting,** and **abdominal pain** (especially in kids). **Coma** can occur without initial medical attention.

Physical findings include **dehydration** (e.g., dry mucous membranes, poor skin turgor, BUN:creatinine ratio > 15:1, hypotension), tachypnea with **rapid deep breathing** due to acidosis (Kussmaul respirations), and a **fruity odor on the breath** (from ketonemia). Diffuse **abdominal tenderness** may be present. Labs reveal **hyperglycemia** (usually > 300 mg/dL), **metabolic acidosis, ketones in the serum and urine, glycosuria, hyponatremia** (from the hyperglycemia), and **elevated serum potassium** (due to cellular shift caused by acidosis, though most patients have a total body potassium deficiency).

Treatment includes **IV fluids, insulin,** and **electrolyte monitoring/ replacement** acutely (especially **potassium,** which usually needs to be given at some point). Once the patient is stabilized, **education, dietary changes, regular insulin,** and close long-term monitoring of glucose control with **hemoglobin A_{1C} levels** (goal is < 7) are needed.

More High-Yield Facts

A "**honeymoon period**" may occur after an initial episode of DKA. This means the patient **no longer needs insulin**. Within a few years the "honeymoon" will end, insulin will be needed, and DM I will be permanent.

Case 47

Internal Medicine

History

A 65-year-old Asian woman is experiencing mid-back pain that started suddenly this morning after she lifted a box of clothes in her basement. The pain is sharp and localized over her spine. She has never had pain like this before. Her past medical history is significant for COPD. Her medications include ipratropium and albuterol metered-dose inhalers, as well as frequent courses of corticosteroids. The patient has smoked for the past 40 years and drinks "several vodka and tonics" per day. She has no children and went through menopause at the age of 45.

Exam

T: 98.6°F BP: 136/84 RR: 16/min. P: 78/min.

The patient is thin and in mild distress secondary to pain. Head, neck, chest, and abdominal exams are unremarkable. The patient has focal tenderness to palpation in the lower thoracic spine. Extremity and neurologic exams are normal.

Tests

Hemoglobin: 15 mg/dL (normal 12–16)
White blood cell count: 8800/μL (normal 4500–11,000)
Platelets: 310,000/μL (normal 150,000–400,000)
Calcium: 9.2 mg/dL (normal 8.5–10.5)
Phosphorus: 3.6 mg/dL (normal 3–4.5)
Thoracic spine x-ray: compression fracture of the T-10 vertebral body
X-ray of hand (from 2 years ago): see figure

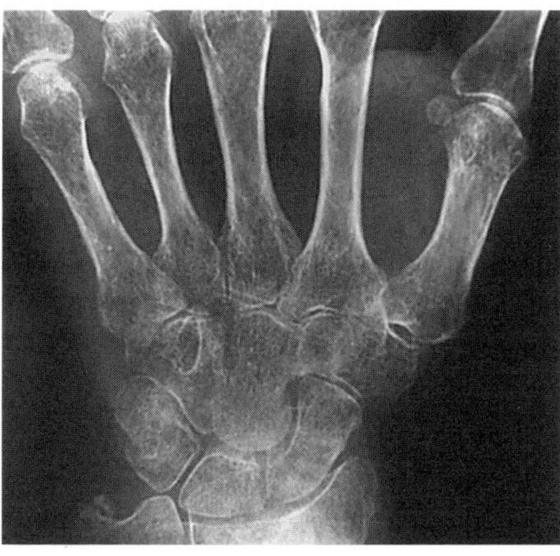

From Katz DS, Math KR, Groskin SA (eds): Radiology Secrets. Philadelphia, Hanley & Belfus, Inc., 1998, pp 257–260; with permission.

Condition Osteoporosis

The hand x-ray reveals marked loss of bone (osteopenia).

Pathophysiology

Osteoporosis is a reduction in the quantity of bone. Most cases are **primary** and thought to be age-related. Risk factors include **increasing age, female sex, thin body habitus, white or Asian race, nulliparity, early menopause, sedentary lifestyle, poor calcium/vitamin D intake, and family history**. Secondary causes include **smoking, alcohol abuse, corticosteroids, hyperparathyroidism, hypogonadism, immobilization, renal failure, malabsorption, COPD,** and liver disease.

The main health risk of osteoporosis is **fractures,** classically of the **hip, vertebral bodies, and wrist**. Roughly **50%** of all women will develop a fracture because of osteoporosis during their lifetime.

Diagnosis & Treatment

Osteoporosis is often asymptomatic until a fracture occurs, usually after a **fall,** though vertebral fractures often occur without trauma. Some patients may complain of **aching pains in the bones,** particularly the back, before a fracture occurs. Vertebral fractures usually cause localized pain that is aggravated by weight bearing.

Findings are limited unless fractures have already occurred. **Kyphosis** (i.e., "hunched back") may occur from multiple vertebral compression fractures. Fractures will generally cause **focal tenderness** to palpation and **limitation of movement**. Calcium, phosphorus, and alkaline phosphatase are **normal**.

The diagnosis can usually be made by x-ray once a fracture has occurred. The bone that is fractured tends to be grossly **demineralized** (i.e., osteopenic). The best time to make the diagnosis, however, is *before* a fracture occurs to allow preventative therapy. **Dual x-ray absorptiometry (DEXA scan)** is commonly used to detect and quantify osteoporosis, which is defined by a bone mineral density (BMD) more than **2.5 standard deviations below the mean** young adult BMD. **Screen** those at high-risk.

Women of all ages should get adequate vitamin D (primarily from **diet** and **sunlight,** need 400 IU/day), calcium (primarily from **dairy** products, with supplements if needed to give women a total of roughly **1000 mg/day**), and **weight-bearing exercise**. Postmenopausal women should be offered **hormone-replacement therapy**. More specific therapies include **bisphosphonates** (e.g., alendronate), intranasal **calcitonin,** and raloxifene.

More High-Yield Facts

Men get osteoporosis, too. Consider screening those at risk.

Case 48

Internal Medicine

History

A 29-year-old man is seeking a second opinion. He says he had a chest x-ray 3 weeks ago for a bout of bronchitis and was told he has a "spot" on his lung. The treating physician told him not to worry about it and said he would check another chest x-ray in several months. The patient has been worried that he may have cancer and wants to know if he needs to have the lesion removed. He has no significant past medical history and takes no medications. The patient does not smoke or use illicit drugs, but drinks alcohol on social occasions. He mentions that his grandfather died of prostate cancer.

Exam

T: 98.6°F BP: 122/78 RR: 12/min. P: 68/min.

The patient is thin and in no acute distress. Head, neck, chest, and abdominal exams are unremarkable. No skin lesions or adenopathy are appreciated. Extremity and neurologic exams are normal.

Tests

Hemoglobin: 16 mg/dL (normal 14–18)
White blood cell count: 6800/μL (normal 4500–11,000)
Platelets: 300,000/μL (normal 150,000–400,000)
X-ray: see figure

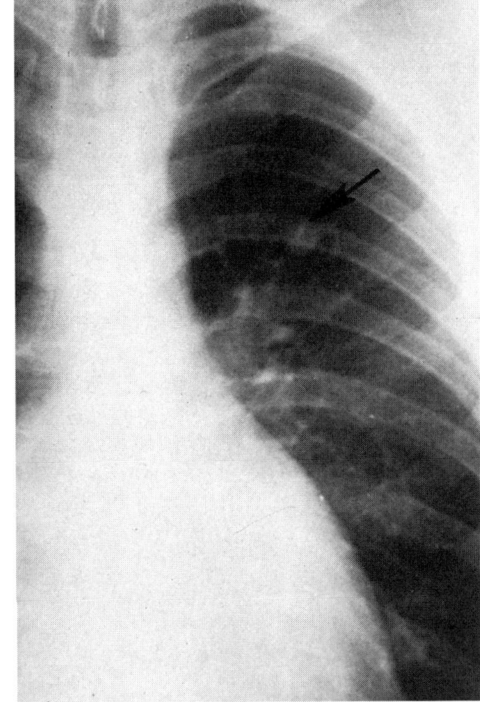

From Juhl JH. In Juhl JH, Crummy AB (eds): Paul and Juhl's Essentials of Radiologic Imaging, 6th ed. Philadelphia, Lippincott, 1993, pp 957–982; with permission.

Condition **Solitary pulmonary nodule (SPN)**

The nodule is shown on the chest x-ray (*arrow*).

Pathophysiology

An SPN is defined as a single, rounded, < **3-cm** diameter density, and is a fairly common diagnostic problem. The primary goal is to characterize the lesion as **benign or malignant**. If this cannot be done radiographically, biopsy or surgical resection is often required. Taking all cases, the risk that an SPN is malignant is about **40%**. However, certain factors can reduce or increase that risk significantly. **Risk factors that favor malignancy include age > 40, smoking history, larger size, irregular margins, and growth over time**. A small SPN in a patient under the age of 30 with no smoking history is malignant in < 5% of cases.

The cause of a benign SPN is usually an **old granuloma** from **tuberculosis** or **fungus** exposure (e.g., *Histoplasma*) or a **hamartoma**.

Diagnosis & Treatment

When an SPN is identified on a chest x-ray, **the first step** in diagnosis is to **look at old chest x-rays or CT scans for comparison**. **If the lesion has not grown in 2 years, it is considered stable** and **can be followed with serial x-rays** every 6 months for another year or two before it is considered almost definitely benign. Additionally, if an SPN is described as having **"popcorn" calcifications** or is completely calcified, it is **usually benign** and can be followed with only repeat chest x-rays every 6 months for 2 years, except in those at extremely high risk for malignancy. If comparison of previous chest x-rays reveals **enlargement of the SPN over time, surgical resection** or biopsy is advisable. **Clinical history** and **findings** also help in the work-up, as a 60-year-old patient who is a heavy smoker with hemoptysis and weight loss will need more aggressive work-up.

If old films are not available and the patient is over age 30 and/or smokes, a **CT scan of the chest** should be performed to evaluate the nodule further and determine if any other nodules or lymphadenopathy is present. If CT cannot characterize the lesion as benign, a **biopsy or surgical resection** of the nodule is advisable in those **over 40**. In a patient under age 40 who doesn't smoke and has no known primary malignancy, an SPN **can be followed with serial chest x-rays or CT scans** every 6 months for 2–3 years to document stability and the presumed benign nature.

More High-Yield Facts

PET scanning is increasingly being used to characterize indeterminate SPNs as benign or malignant and has a low false-negative rate (doesn't miss cancer), though false-positives may occur (e.g., active granulomas).

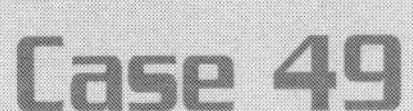

Internal Medicine

History

A 24-year-old woman presents to the emergency department (ED) with a chief complaint of severe chest pain and shortness of breath. She says she feels as though she is going to die. The patient also reports sweating and feels her heart beating "like crazy." Her symptoms all began suddenly roughly 20 minutes ago. She was in the ED 1 week ago with similar complaints, and no cause could be found for her symptoms. Past medical history is otherwise unremarkable, and the patient takes no regular medications. She does not smoke, drink alcohol, or use illicit drugs. Family history is notable for paternal hypertension.

Exam

T: 98.8°F BP: 132/84 RR: 20/min. P: 98/min.

The patient is markedly tachypneic and anxious. Her skin is clammy, but good skin turgor is present. Head, neck, and lung exams are unremarkable. Cardiac exam reveals borderline tachycardia and a mid-systolic click followed by a late-systolic soft murmur. Abdominal, pelvic, rectal, extremity, and neurologic exams are normal.

Tests

Hemoglobin: 14 mg/dL (normal 12–16)
White blood cell count: 7000/μL (normal 4500–11,000)
Platelets: 320,000/μL (normal 150,000–400,000)
Sodium: 140 meq/L (normal 135–145)
Potassium: 4 meq/L (normal 3.5–5)
Creatinine: 1 mg/dL (normal 0.6–1.5)
Thyroid-stimulating hormone: 2.2 μU/mL (normal 0.5–5)
Erythrocyte sedimentation rate: 8 mm/hr (normal 1–20)
Creatine phosphokinase: 32 u/L (normal 17–148)
Chest x-ray: normal
24-hour urine for vanillylmandelic acid: normal
Arterial blood gases: pH: 7.48
pO_2: 108 torr (normal 80–100)
pCO_2: 30 mmHg (normal 35–45)
HCO_3^-: 26 meq/L
EKG: see figure

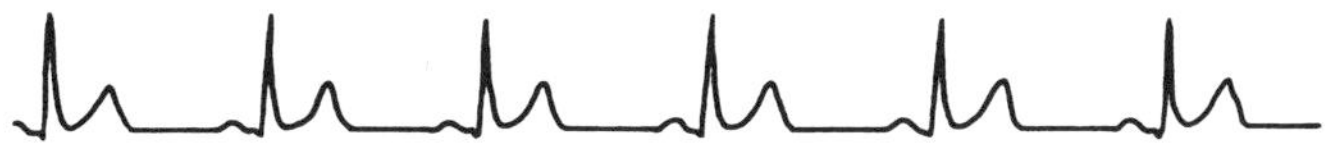

From Wolf PS, Giugliano GR: Cardiovascular physical diagnosis. In Adair OV (ed): Cardiology Secrets, 2nd ed. Philadelphia, Hanley & Belfus, Inc. 2001, pp 1–7; with permission.

Condition Panic disorder

The EKG shows a **normal sinus rhythm** with no abnormalities.

Pathophysiology

Panic disorder consists of recurrent **panic attacks,** which are a manifestation of anxiety. This disorder occurs with agoraphobia roughly 50% of the time. The etiology is uncertain, but there is a definite **genetic component** and a classic association with **mitral valve prolapse**. The disorder often presents **before the age of 30.**

Diagnosis & Treatment

Symptoms may include any of the following: **palpitations, sweating, trembling/ shaking, shortness of breath, a feeling of choking, chest pain/ discomfort, nausea or abdominal pain, dizziness or lightheadedness, fear of losing control/ going crazy, fear of dying,** a feeling of unreality (**derealization**), and a feeling of being detached from oneself (**depersonalization**). **At least four** of these symptoms should be present, and the symptoms should occur **suddenly** and **peak within 10 minutes**. A history of prior attacks without a discovered cause is common. The dramatic symptoms can mimic a **myocardial infarction, arrhythmia, pheochromocytoma,** and **hyperthyroidism,** which should all be ruled out.

Physical findings are related to extreme anxiety: **hypertension, tachypnea** (a **primary respiratory alkalosis** without metabolic compensation, as in this case, is generally present), **tachycardia,** and **diaphoresis**. The **murmur** of mitral valve prolapse may be present (as in this case). On Step 2, all tests and lab values given in the question will be *normal.*

Treatment includes psychotherapy, usually a form of **cognitive behavioral therapy,** and **medications**. The preferred first-line agent is a **serotonin-selective reuptake inhibitor (SSRI),** such as fluoxetine. Other effective agents include **benzodiazepines** (addictive potential) and tricyclic antidepressants or monoamine-oxidase inhibitors (both have less favorable side-effect profiles compared to SSRIs).

More High-Yield Facts

Agoraphobia is anxiety about being in **certain places or situations** because the person fears having a panic attack. Those affected usually prefer to **stay in their home** and/or **avoid crowded situations** or places that don't allow an easy escape (e.g., riding on a bus). If necessary, such places/situations are **endured with extreme anxiety**. Often, affected persons require a **companion** to go with them. Treatment is generally similar to panic disorder without agoraphobia.

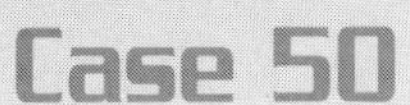

Case 50

Internal Medicine

History

A 48-year-old woman presents for a routine office visit. She was diagnosed with type II diabetes mellitus at her last visit 1 month ago and was started on metformin. The patient reports no significant side effects from the medications and says she feels much better since the last time she saw you. She tells you that she plans to follow all of your instructions and wants to be in the best health she can be. The patient asks what the best ways are to monitor her diabetes. She also wants information about specific health risks. She has no other medical problems and takes no other medications.

Exam

T: 98.5°F BP: 132/84 RR: 140/min. P: 68/min.

The patient is slightly overweight. Her funduscopic exam reveals no apparent abnormalities. Cardiac exam is normal. Neurologic exam reveals normal vibratory sense in all extremities. The rest of the exam is also normal. What diabetes-specific treatments, monitoring, and preventive care would you recommend?

Tests

Hemoglobin: 14 mg/dL (normal 12–16)
Creatinine: 1 mg/dL (normal 0.6–1.5)
BUN: 12 mg/dL (normal 8–25)
Glucose, fasting: 105 mg/dL (normal fasting 70–110)
Urinalysis: 1+ protein; negative for glucose, bacteria, and white blood cells

Issue

Routine care and preventive health for diabetes mellitus (DM)

Pathophysiology

As discussed in previous cases, DM can cause multiple short-term and long-term health risks. Management of these issues is a common clinical situation, and you should understand the basics before taking Step 2.

Diagnosis & Treatment

Once a diagnosis of type II DM is made, the following are part of routine care for life:

• Glucose: patients should monitor their levels **daily,** preferably three times a day, and keep a written log of the values. In addition, you should measure the glucose and **hemoglobin A_{1c}** (goal of < 7) at least annually and more often in cases with poor control and after medication changes. If insulin is used, know how to adjust either NPH or regular insulin doses. If **7 AM** glucose is high (low), increase (decrease) **NPH insulin** at dinner the night before. If **noon** glucose is high (low), increase (decrease) **morning regular insulin**. If **5 PM** glucose is high (low), increase (decrease) **morning NPH insulin**. If **9 PM** glucose is high (low), increase (decrease) dinner-time **regular insulin**.

• Kidney dysfunction: monitor for **microalbuminuria** at least annually. If it develops, put the patient on an **ACE-inhibitor,** which delays progression of renal disease. The patient in this case likely needs an ACE-inhibitor. Be very careful giving patients with diabetes **IV contrast agents** (e.g., for a CT scan or intravenous pyelogram) if they have evidence of renal insufficiency. If IV contrast is required, use **generous IV hydration** immediately prior to and after the contrast is given to avoid renal damage.

• Retinopathy: at diagnosis, a **baseline ophthalmology exam** is recommended. Re-examination every 6 months to 2 years based on the status of diabetic eye disease is needed. **Panretinal photocoagulation** is done for **proliferative retinopathy** (i.e., neovascularization).

• Neuropathy: distal lower extremities should be examined at least annually with a **thin monofilament** to test for sensory/position loss. If present, special **foot care** is required, including wearing of comfortable, properly fitting shoes and patient **self-foot inspection** on a daily basis.

• Cardiovascular disease: other atherosclerosis risk factors need to be **screened for and managed aggressively if found,** including smoking, cholesterol, and hypertension.

More High-Yield Facts

Always encourage **regular exercise** and a **healthy diet** with avoidance of high-carbohydrate foods. **Weight loss** often reduces the need for medications and in some cases can reverse overt diabetes entirely.

CASE INDEX

Notes

Notes

Notes

Notes

Notes

Notes

Notes

Notes

Notes

Notes

Notes

Notes

Notes

Notes

Notes

Notes

Notes

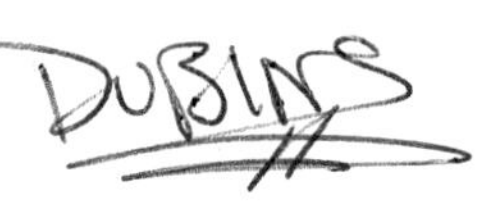

Notes

Bruce Stress test protocol

Stage 1	3 min	10% incline	1.7 mph	4.7 mets
Stage 2	6 min	12% "	2.5 mph	7.0 "
Stage 3	9 min	14% "	3.4 mph	10.1 "
Stage 4	12 min	16% "	4.2 mph	12.9 "
Stage 5	15 min	18% "	5.0 mph	15.0 "

nml

I ↑	aVR	V_1	V_4
II	aVL	V_2	V_5
III	aVF ↑	V_3	V_6

nml

I ↑	aVR	V_1	V_4
II ↑	aVL	V_2	V_5
III	aVF ↓	V_3	V_6

Rt deviation

I ↓	aVR	V_1	V_4
II	aVL	V_2	V_5
III	aVF ↑	V_3	V_6

Lt De

I ↑	aVR	V_1	V_4
II ↓	aVL	V_2	V_5
II	aVF ↓	V_3	V_6

① Long PR interval = 1st Degree ♡ Block

②

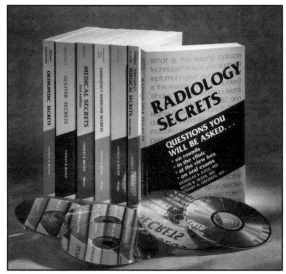

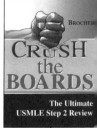

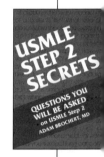

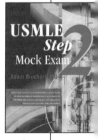

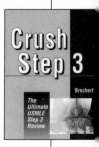